52-WEEK GRIEF JOURNAL

52-WEEK grief journal

PROMPTS AND REFLECTIONS FOR NAVIGATING LOSS

JENNIFER TRINKLE, LMFT

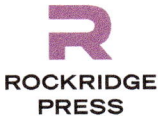

ROCKRIDGE PRESS

Copyright © 2022 by Rockridge Press, Oakland, California

No part of this publication may be reproduced, stored in a retrieval system, or transmitted in any form or by any means, electronic, mechanical, photocopying, recording, scanning, or otherwise, except as permitted under Sections 107 or 108 of the 1976 United States Copyright Act, without the prior written permission of the Publisher. Requests to the Publisher for permission should be addressed to the Permissions Department, Rockridge Press, 1955 Broadway, Suite 400, Oakland, CA 94612.

Limit of Liability/Disclaimer of Warranty: The Publisher and the author make no representations or warranties with respect to the accuracy or completeness of the contents of this work and specifically disclaim all warranties, including without limitation warranties of fitness for a particular purpose. No warranty may be created or extended by sales or promotional materials. The advice and strategies contained herein may not be suitable for every situation. This work is sold with the understanding that the Publisher is not engaged in rendering medical, legal, or other professional advice or services. If professional assistance is required, the services of a competent professional person should be sought. Neither the Publisher nor the author shall be liable for damages arising herefrom. The fact that an individual, organization, or website is referred to in this work as a citation and/or potential source of further information does not mean that the author or the Publisher endorses the information the individual, organization, or website may provide or recommendations they/it may make. Further, readers should be aware that websites listed in this work may have changed or disappeared between when this work was written and when it is read.

For general information on our other products and services or to obtain technical support, please contact our Customer Care Department within the United States at (866) 744-2665, or outside the United States at (510) 253-0500.

Rockridge Press publishes its books in a variety of electronic and print formats. Some content that appears in print may not be available in electronic books, and vice versa.

TRADEMARKS: Rockridge Press and the Rockridge Press logo are trademarks or registered trademarks of Callisto Media Inc. and/or its affiliates, in the United States and other countries, and may not be used without written permission. All other trademarks are the property of their respective owners. Rockridge Press is not associated with any product or vendor mentioned in this book.

Interior and Cover Designer: Helen Bruno
Art Producer: Alyssa Williams
Editor: Brian Sweeting
Production Editor: Emily Sheehan
Production Manager: Riley Hoffman

Illustrations © Microvector/Creative Market; Author photo courtesy of Elizabeth Dixon

Paperback ISBN: 978-1-63878-091-5
R0

This journal belongs to:

....

CONTENTS

INTRODUCTION..x

HOW TO USE THIS JOURNAL...xii

WEEK 1: You Are Where You Need to Be...1

WEEK 2: Thawing Emotional Numbness..4

WEEK 3: Honoring Your Anger..8

WEEK 4: Releasing Your Guilt..11

WEEK 5: Identifying Grief in Your Body..14

WEEK 6: Creating New Expectations...18

WEEK 7: Accepting Your Uncertainty..21

WEEK 8: Navigating the Fog of Grief..24

WEEK 9: Healthy and Unhealthy Ways of Coping..............................27

WEEK 10: Exhaustion and the Need to Rest.......................................31

WEEK 11: The Loneliness of Absence...34

WEEK 12: Feeling Abandoned..37

- **WEEK 13:** Acknowledging Despair ... 40
- **WEEK 14:** Coming to Terms with Changing Responsibilities ... 43
- **WEEK 15:** Choosing Rituals and Practices to Mark Your Loss ... 47
- **WEEK 16:** Handling Other Peoples' Expectations ... 50
- **WEEK 17:** Finding Meaning Through Tears ... 53
- **WEEK 18:** Facing Reminders ... 56
- **WEEK 19:** Feeling Like No One Understands ... 59
- **WEEK 20:** The Burden of Regret ... 62
- **WEEK 21:** Finding Yourself Again ... 65
- **WEEK 22:** Sitting with Unresolved, Prolonged, or Complicated Grief ... 68
- **WEEK 23:** Making Decisions, Big and Little ... 71
- **WEEK 24:** Am I Grieving, Depressed, or Both? ... 74
- **WEEK 25:** Acknowledging Stuck Points ... 78
- **WEEK 26:** Mourning Intimacy and Connection ... 81

WEEK 27:	**Your Feelings About Changing Relationships**	84
WEEK 28:	**Honoring Your Loved One**	87
WEEK 29:	**Accepting the Passage of Time**	90
WEEK 30:	**Finding Your People**	94
WEEK 31:	**Transcending Loss Through Creativity, Art, and Music**	97
WEEK 32:	**Gathering Your Memories**	100
WEEK 33:	**Keeping Connected to Your Loved One**	103
WEEK 34:	**Looking for Signs**	106
WEEK 35:	**Anticipating Birthdays, Anniversaries, and Holidays**	109
WEEK 36:	**Nurturing Hope**	112
WEEK 37:	**Recognizing Sudden Bouts of Grief**	115
WEEK 38:	**What I Didn't Expect About Grief**	118
WEEK 39:	**The Many Meanings of Afterlife**	122
WEEK 40:	**Love Survives Loss**	125

WEEK 41: Cultivating Gratitude	128
WEEK 42: Opening Up About Grief	131
WEEK 43: The Importance of Showing Up	134
WEEK 44: Finding Strength in Yourself and Others	137
WEEK 45: Handling the Permanence of Loss	141
WEEK 46: Creating Meaning and Finding Purpose	144
WEEK 47: Giving Back	148
WEEK 48: Checking in with Where You Are Now	151
WEEK 49: Finding Comfort in Beauty	154
WEEK 50: Recognizing Your Inner Strength	157
WEEK 51: What Does It Mean to Heal?	160
WEEK 52: Visualizing the Future	164
RESOURCES	168

INTRODUCTION

YOU ARE HERE because you have experienced a profound loss and want to make sense of it. You are not alone in this journey. Grief is universal, an essential part of being human. Your deep sadness is a testament to your capacity to love. But with connection eventually comes the inevitable pain of loss. Often, grief is complicated—because our relationships are complicated. Long illnesses, unexpected deaths, unfinished business, or unresolved conflicts affect how we grieve. The other emotions that emerge, such as guilt, anger, and regret, are totally normal and encouraging signs that you are human.

My own experiences with grief are many, including the deaths of grandparents, my mother's longtime partner, and too many pets to count. But nothing prepared me for my father's death from an aggressive brain tumor. The tumor robbed him of the capacity to walk or speak. My father's wit, attention to detail, and warm curiosity were taken before he was physically gone. Grieving started with his illness.

After coming out of the initial shock of my father's rapid decline and death, the first weeks were the hardest, a blur of numbness, disbelief, guilt, and sadness. His death left me empty. I missed Dad's engaged conversation and cut-to-the-chase attitude. Aching for his presence, I sought comfort in signs and dreams, connections from beyond.

Sharing memories with my mother and stepmother and writing about my dad helped me process my loss. Having gratitude for the relationship we created in the years before his death was also healing. I've learned that my father lives within me. I can summon his voice and anticipate his advice even in his absence. The raw, ragged waves of early grief have mainly subsided, though they return from time to time.

This journal is for anyone who is grieving and wants guidance and tools to work through their feelings. Having a space to reflect helps create order out of grief's chaos. As you get words down on paper, a story will emerge; as you preserve memories, you will discover new ways of seeing the past. In addition, mindful reflection and thinking concretely about self-care can help you feel grounded in a time when so much is unclear.

If your relationship with your loved one was difficult or unresolved, you may come to this book with complicated feelings. The loss of someone we had a problematic relationship with, such as an estranged child, ex-partner, or abusive family member, is particularly thorny. Traumatic losses through violence, suicide, or substance use are also difficult to come to terms with. Mourning someone who is still physically present, but feels gone because of a degenerative disease or a severe, persistent mental illness, can bring up complex feelings. Similarly, we may struggle when we experience grief in anticipation of a loved one's death. This journal helps you untangle your emotions and create meaning out of them.

Grieving permeates every aspect of life. It makes socializing feel impossible. Concentration and the ability to think clearly go missing. We eat too much and can't seem to sleep, or eat too little and can't seem to stop sleeping. Be kind to yourself as you go through this period of upheaval. With time and space, the ache of grief will become less intense.

HOW TO USE THIS JOURNAL

GRIEF DOESN'T FOLLOW A SCHEDULE. Just as there is no right or wrong way to grieve, there is no right or wrong way to use this journal. Feel free to move around the entries according to what is most pressing for you in the moment. Let the journal be an open and friendly space where you freely jot down whatever comes to mind without judgment or censorship.

Each week has a different grief-related theme and is divided into six days, with a built-in day off. To help you stay grounded and set positive, compassionate intentions for the days ahead, every week starts with an affirmation. This is followed by four prompts and an exercise designed to deepen your thinking, remember your loved one, and connect with your feelings. Some prompts and exercises focus on self-care. When the week is done, allow yourself that day of rest. Although grief doesn't take a break, it is important to give yourself a break from introspection. Simply feeling what you feel, without making sense of it, is an essential part of healing.

Although the weekly format suggests an order, you can start this journal at whatever place makes sense for you right now. If a prompt or exercise doesn't feel useful, skipping it and returning to it later is totally fine. Perhaps you want to start by working through feelings of guilt (Releasing Your Guilt, Week 4) or are worried about how you will handle an upcoming significant date (Anticipating Birthdays, Anniversaries, and Holidays, Week 35). For readers who are feeling alone with their grief, I recommend starting with Week 11 (The Loneliness of Absence) or Week 19 (Feeling Like No One Understands). As you work through the journal, you can also look back at past entries to see how your perspective has shifted.

This book is not a substitute for professional treatment. Distinguishing depression from grief can be tricky. Grief allows for an ebb and flow of emotion and is focused on the loss. Depression is all-encompassing and centered on negative feelings about the self. Pay attention to the intensity, persistence, and focus of your feelings. If hopelessness and despair continue or intensify, or if you are feeling worthless, continue to struggle with eating and sleeping, or are seriously considering suicide, please seek professional support.

Even if you aren't struggling with mental health, talking with a professional can help. Meeting one-on-one with a psychotherapist or joining a group of other grieving folks can lessen feelings of loneliness and deepen connection. I've included a list of resources at the end of the book.

WEEK 1

You Are Where You Need to Be

MY GRIEF HAS NO SCHEDULE. I AM
WHERE I NEED TO BE AT THIS MOMENT.

Sometimes others expect us to be "over" our loss quickly. They might ask why we haven't snapped out of our sadness or tell us everyone dies, with the implication we should be able to easily let go of our loved ones. These messages are easy to internalize, in addition to being irritating or even infuriating. Imagine you could respond however you wished, without filter, to people who pressure you to be past your grief. What would you say? What emotions arise?

Grief experts Elisabeth Kübler-Ross and David Kessler identified five "stages" of grief: denial, anger, bargaining, depression, and acceptance. These stages can be experienced—and reexperienced—at any time in the grieving process. There is no right order or absolute end point. What stage are you at today? Where were you last week?

_____
_____
_____
_____
_____
_____

Grief varies in intensity from week to week and month to month. Think about the feelings that make up your grief. How would you represent each feeling in color? For example, you might use deep purple for the saddest days, fire-engine red for anger, and beige for the blahs. What color is your grief today?

_____
_____
_____
_____
_____
_____

Many of us carry around the burden of "shoulds," or things we believe we *should* have done, words we *should* have said. These beliefs interfere with our capacity to process our grief. What beliefs do you have about where you should be in terms of your grief? What influences those beliefs?

_____
_____
_____
_____
_____
_____
_____
_____

VISUALIZE RELEASE

Sit in a relaxed, comfortable position. Close your eyes. Breathe in and out slowly, letting your breath fall into a steady, even rhythm. Picture those "shoulds," each dense and heavy as a brick, filling a shopping bag. Imagine you are walking down a sidewalk carrying this bag of beliefs. The bag's straps cut into your hands. Your feet are tired, and your shoulders ache. You notice a trash can coming up and decide you have carried this burden long enough. One by one you let the beliefs fall into the trash, each landing with a satisfying thud. You feel immediate relief. Rub your shoulders. Shake out your hands. Take a few moments to relish the feeling of lightness before opening your eyes.

WEEK 2

Thawing Emotional Numbness

THIS NUMBNESS IS TEMPORARY. I TRUST MY MIND AND BODY TO PROTECT ME AND GET ME THROUGH THIS DIFFICULT TIME.

Feeling numb is a stress response. It serves a purpose, allowing us to be somewhat functional in the aftermath of terrible things. It keeps our hearts from collapsing with the grief and protects our capacity to think. Are there aspects of feeling numb you appreciate? How does your numbness protect you?

When our feelings of despair are dulled, our feelings of joy and connection are blunted as well. This can be scary. We feel cut off from a part of ourselves, worried that we will never feel anything again. Do you have these worries? What parts of you are dulled by numbness?

Our numbness can feel like several layers of padding between us and our emotions. Protected from pain, we also struggle to move and feel freely. At some point, the muffling of feeling is too restrictive. We need to remove a layer or two. What would it look like to shed a layer of your numbness? How would you feel?

Have you ever been so cold you've lost feeling in your fingers or toes? It is an unsettling, and sometimes dangerous, experience. If we stay cold too long, we can develop frostbite. As our body warms, our skin tingles and burns. It hurts. Something similar happens when our emotional numbness starts to thaw. What might you feel as your numbness recedes?

DO A TASK MINDFULLY

When we feel emotionally numb, doing routine activities mindfully grounds us in the present. The key is to slow down and pay attention to our senses, taking in what we hear, see, smell, touch, and taste. Pick a task you do regularly, such as washing the dishes, making and drinking coffee, or folding laundry. Make an intention to focus totally on this task while you are doing it.

> **Sometimes taking this mindful approach can feel too intense. If you find yourself becoming overwhelmed, stop. Write down how you felt before and then after this mindful practice.**

WEEK 3

Honoring Your Anger

**I HONOR MY ANGER AND ALLOW
MYSELF SPACE TO EXPRESS IT SAFELY.**

Anger is a common reaction to loss. The force of our anger can frighten or embarrass us. Sometimes it makes us feel guilty. Being angry can also seem useless. (It won't bring our loved ones back.) Our beliefs about anger and the "right" way to express it are affected by cultural expectations and how our families handled anger growing up. What beliefs do you have about anger? How do they affect your grief?

We may blame our loved ones for leaving us, for not taking better care of themselves, for making fatal mistakes; or, we are angry at those responsible for their deaths. This is normal. We have the right to feel angry, even when the focus of our anger is dead. What has grief made you furious about?

Our anger is sometimes a cover for other emotions, such as fear or sadness. When we don't acknowledge or process those underlying feelings, they can come out as anger. As you grieve, what other emotions might be underneath your anger?

When anger doesn't have an outlet, it can turn into rage. Rage incites us to do and say things we regret. Catching the physical signs of anger early can interrupt the process. Fueled by adrenaline, our heart rates increase. Our jaws clench. We feel hot. Sometimes we tremble. How does anger show up in your body?

EXPRESS ANGER SAFELY

Anger and rage burn us from the inside out. They often end up directed at innocent targets, such as unhelpful customer service representatives or clueless friends and family members. Spouting off feels good in the moment but can hurt others and doesn't erase the underlying feeling. Give voice to your anger and rage in a way that creates no victims. Grab a stack of blank pieces of paper. Write out your angry grief thoughts, one per sheet. Take it out on the page. Be ugly. Be brutal. Scribble. Use all caps. Crumple up those pages one by one and throw them against a wall until your anger feels appeased.

Releasing Your Guilt

I RELEASE MY GUILT AROUND MY LOVED ONE AND THEIR DEATH AND ALLOW MYSELF FORGIVENESS AND LIGHT.

Our guilt feels vast. There are things we wish we had never said or done. We feel guilty for the moments we forget our loved ones or when we're angry with them or relieved they're gone. Writing down these feelings releases some of their power. What guilt do you carry around your loss?

_____
_____
_____
_____
_____
_____
_____
_____
_____
_____

The past cannot be changed. Continuing to focus on past mistakes keeps guilt alive. In a way, this focus keeps the dead alive as well, keeps our connection fresh. Letting go of guilt can feel like letting go of our loved ones. What would it mean to release your guilt?

_____

_____

_____

_____

_____

_____

Our dead are no longer here. The present does not affect them. Still, we feel conflicted about living our lives fully after their loss. Happy moments lead to guilty ones, as though our loved ones would expect us to exist in constant sadness. Moments of forgetting feel like betrayal. What would it be like to allow yourself happiness without guilt?

_____

_____

_____

_____

_____

_____

Engaging with our guilt and providing it with counterevidence gives us a more realistic sense of culpability. For example, I felt guilty I did not visit my father and stepmother the last Christmas my father was alive. I ease my guilt by reminding myself that no one knew he had brain cancer or expected him to be dead in two months. What counterevidence do you have against your guilt?

___

ASK FORGIVENESS

This psychotherapy technique can be used to ask forgiveness from your loved one. Sit facing an empty chair. In the chair, picture the person you have lost. Speak to them, outlining what you feel guilty about and where you would like their forgiveness or acceptance. When you are done, move to the empty chair and speak from your loved one's point of view. Move between positions until your feelings are more resolved. Return to this technique if guilt reemerges or you need to work something out.

What was this exercise like for you? Did anything shift?

WEEK 5

Identifying Grief in Your Body

MY PHYSICAL AND MENTAL HEALTH ARE IMPORTANT. I PLEDGE TO TAKE CARE OF MYSELF AND GET HELP WHEN I NEED IT.

Grief stresses our bodies and our minds. We need time to take care of our health but often lack the capacity or desire to focus on ourselves. With our loved ones gone, our health no longer feels important. What gets in the way of taking care of yourself?

We hold grief in different places in our bodies. For example, after my father died, my body was keyed up and my mind filled with racing thoughts and worries. My appetite and sleep fell away. I also had a hard time thinking clearly. How does grief show up in your body?

If our loved ones suffered or were ill before dying, it can affect how we approach our own health. For example, we may feel guilty about self-care or avoid health care settings because of their traumatic associations. Or we may become anxious about potential symptoms. Have your attitudes toward your physical or mental health been affected by your loved one's suffering? If so, how?

Identifying Grief in Your Body

Grief depletes our energy and robs us of vitality. Stress hormones course through our bodies, affecting our physical and mental health. Because of this extra load, being deliberate about our self-care can help us stay as healthy as possible. What are you doing to take special care of yourself as you grieve?

PAY ATTENTION TO YOUR SYMPTOMS

Grief is associated with multiple physical and psychological symptoms. Some of these are more serious than others. Items marked in bold merit the immediate attention of a health care or mental health professional. Check off what you have experienced after loss. If any symptoms persist for more than a few weeks, seek out professional support with someone sensitive to the needs of grievers.

PHYSICAL SYMPTOMS

- ☐ **Chest pain**
- ☐ **Shortness of breath**
- ☐ Headaches
- ☐ Dry mouth
- ☐ Insomnia
- ☐ Nausea
- ☐ Stomach pain
- ☐ Decreased appetite
- ☐ Fatigue
- ☐ Muscle soreness

PSYCHOLOGICAL SYMPTOMS

- ☐ **Persistent, intense sadness**
- ☐ **Panic attacks**
- ☐ **Excessive worry**
- ☐ **Difficulty concentrating**
- ☐ **Forgetfulness and brain fog**
- ☐ **Social withdrawal**
- ☐ **Irritability**

WEEK 6

Creating New Expectations

LIVING WITH THE REALITY OF DEATH TAKES BRAVERY. ON DAYS WHEN I FEEL LESS BRAVE, I KNOW MY COURAGE WILL RETURN.

Denial is a defense mechanism, a way our unconscious protects us from becoming overwhelmed. It can be a healthy way to cope in hard times. Denying reality completely or for too long, however, causes trouble. How do you use denial to cope? When is it healthy? When could it be harmful?

Though denial can be pleasant and sometimes necessary, denying the reality of loss creates false hope. Accepting the way things are makes space for realistic expectations. To cultivate hope based in reality, it helps to identify what is truly real and possible, optimism grounded in fact.

People who expect us to quickly be "over" a loss are in denial. Although others ignore the cruel truth of death, we can't escape it. But we were once just like them. Their denial is temporary and protective: Everyone eventually experiences loss. What has grief brought that you wish you could deny?

More than once, I've passed someone on the street who resembles my mother's long-dead partner. For a brief, lovely moment, I picture him alive, existing in the world. It doesn't even matter that he hasn't been in touch for two decades. I'm just happy that he still exists. This short, fantastical foray into denial brings me comfort. How does denial comfort you?

CHECK IN WITH YOUR LOVED ONE

You are not in denial. Your loved one exists within you. You hold their mannerisms. You sometimes hear their voice in your head, giving advice, pronouncing judgment, or professing love. You might have half of their DNA. Sometimes what you carry of them is invisible, such as an assured sense of self, a struggle to be vulnerable, or a need for control. You know them from the inside out. Conjure them up. Tell them of your struggles with grief. Ask for advice on living without them. What do they say?

WEEK 7

Accepting Your Uncertainty

WITH LOSS COMES CHANGE AND UNCERTAINTY. IT IS NORMAL TO FEEL ANXIOUS AND AFRAID. I CAN HANDLE THIS.

Loss creates practical concerns and amorphous anxieties. Finances change. Responsibilities shift. These are problems that usually can be solved. Anxiety comes with worries that have no solution. Naming our concerns and anxieties helps us tell the difference. What are your concerns? What are your anxieties? (For example, a concern may be finding child care, and an anxiety could be worrying you will never love again.)

Suppressed emotions sometimes show up as anxiety. Becoming aware of these underlying feelings and expressing them openly can help soothe our anxious minds. In grief, these underground emotions could include sadness, anger, guilt, and loneliness, among others. What emotions might be underneath your anxiety?

After a death, the path ahead is unclear. Fear of the unknown is paralyzing. We rebuild our lives one step at a time, using daily goals as guideposts. These goals can be as simple as eating and showering every day. Create a few daily goals to ground you when life is uncertain.

Grief drops us into a new, bleak landscape. What once was simple becomes terrifying. Breaking down overwhelming tasks makes them feel possible. For example, if seeing a friend is too much, text or call them. Name one thing you are afraid to do. Can you break it down into small steps?

PRACTICE 4-7-8 BREATHING

When anxiety is overwhelming, 4-7-8 breathing calms our frazzled minds and bodies. In this breathing exercise, not only is the exhale slightly longer than the inhale, but there is a long pause between them. If this breathing exercise is challenging, shorten the intervals, keeping the ratio (for example, 2-3.5-4).

Sit in a comfortable position. Close your eyes if you wish. Inhale through your nose slowly to the count of four, letting your abdomen expand with your breath, directing the air to your belly and not your chest. Hold your breath for seven seconds, then exhale out your mouth to the count of eight by pursing your lips and making a whooshing sound. In this exhale, push the breath out by tightening your stomach and pulling your diaphragm toward your spine. Repeat up to four times a session. Do this twice a day for maximum benefit.

WEEK 8

Navigating the Fog of Grief

I AM GRIEVING. MY MIND AND HEART ARE STILL PROCESSING MY LOSS. AFTER THIS CONFUSION WILL COME NEW UNDERSTANDING.

The confusion of grief resembles the deep fog of depression. Preoccupied with loss, unable to think straight, we absentmindedly repeat mistakes. Sometimes the fog is so thick we're not even aware of our stumbles. We fall down and lurch forward, never noticing the bruises. How has the fog of grief affected you?

When nothing makes sense, a routine provides predictability. Having a regular schedule keeps us from flying off the edges of the earth. Consistent bed and waking times as well as regular meals are good starting points, even when sleep and appetite feel elusive. Write a few simple, achievable daily goals for yourself.

Some days are just going to be a muddle. Grief is at the helm, using up our capacity to think. Focusing on a meditative activity, such as drawing or yoga, is soothing. What do you do when your mind is fogged in?

Many responsibilities, such as going to work or parenting, are not optional. But if we don't get a break, our confusion can deepen, sometimes leading us to make dangerous mistakes. Whom can you call on for respite when you need to take care of business but are having trouble focusing?

_____
_____
_____
_____
_____
_____
_____

FOCUS ON KNOTS

Grief leaves our minds tied up in knots. But knots are not always illogical tangles of string. They can be tidy, organized ways to keep things secure. Knots serve a purpose. This time of confusion also has a purpose. It creates space to concentrate on grieving.

The process of making knots can be engrossing and helps with focus. Start with a simple square knot. Cross two pieces of string or yarn, one under the other, to make a half knot, as though you were starting to tie a shoe. Cross them a second time, in the opposite order, to form a symmetrical, square knot. Repeat as necessary. To move on to more complicated knots, look at the website Animated Knots (animatedknots.com). If knots aren't your thing, braiding (and unbraiding) are excellent substitutes.

WEEK 9

Healthy and Unhealthy Ways of Coping

I CAN HANDLE GRIEF. I CHOOSE HEALTHY WAYS TO COPE AND DESERVE NOURISHING FOOD, A GOOD NIGHT'S REST, AND COMPASSION.

Death overwhelms some families. Others never speak of the dead again. When emotions feel boundless or inexpressible, they become terrifying. We avoid them through alcohol, drugs, food, or compulsive behaviors. What lessons did you learn when growing up about coping with loss?

After a death, escape becomes appealing. It is a natural, human response to want to dull the pain. Often our attempts to escape provide relief in the moment, but the underlying pain remains. How do you cope with the pain of grief? Where might you need support around coping?

_____
_____
_____
_____
_____
_____

Grief isolates us. In our isolation, we turn to unhealthy ways of coping to cover over our sadness. We also lack energy to try something different. Learning new things activates our brains, expanding our ways of coping. How do you feel about learning something new? What would you be interested in learning?

_____
_____
_____
_____
_____
_____

It is very common to hide our less healthy ways of coping. We may feel embarrassed, ashamed, and alone. Being kind to ourselves around the various ways we cope can help us open up and seek support if we need it. Write an understanding note to the part of you that wants to numb the pain, acknowledging its desire to protect you from hurt. If you think you would benefit from professional support around coping, turn to the Resources section at the end of the book.

MAKE A SELF-CARE PLAN

Taking care of ourselves requires planning. Mark your intentions for self-care. Use the blank lines to create your own goals.

I WILL STRIVE TO:

☐ Eat three nutritious meals a day

☐ Get at least seven hours of sleep a night, going to sleep by _____ and waking up by _____

☐ Move my body at least once a day by _____ or by _____

☐ Reach out to a friend (Who? _____)

☐ Bathe regularly

☐ Take breaks when I need them

☐ Forgive myself when I make mistakes or backslide

☐ _____

☐ _____

☐ _____

I WILL AVOID:

☐ Excessive drinking or drug use (defined as: _____)

☐ Eating foods that are not good for my body, such as _____

☐ Not allowing myself enough time to sleep

☐ _____

☐ _____

☐ _____

☐ _____

WEEK 10

Exhaustion and the Need to Rest

**I AM COPING WITH A LOSS. MY ENERGY WILL RETURN.
I HONOR MY NEED FOR REST AND SLOWNESS.**

Interacting with people feels exhausting. They ask questions we can't easily answer ("How are you doing?"). They expect us to be who we used to be. In protecting them from our grief, we often burden ourselves. Think of a recent frustrating interaction. What did you say? What did you want to say?

Grief is relentless. It drains us of energy and motivation. But sometimes our exhaustion comes from doing too much. We may have returned to our responsibilities prematurely. We may need more time to just be. Taking that time and reducing our task load can bring up both relief and guilt. What gets in the way of giving yourself a break?

_____
_____
_____
_____
_____
_____

When coping with the bone-deep tiredness of grief, we sometimes need time to sit with our feelings or simply be alone. Withdrawing briefly from social obligations is the right thing to do. Sometimes this solitary time becomes exhausting, and we get trapped in isolation. What do you need right now? Is your time alone rejuvenating or contributing to exhaustion?

_____
_____
_____
_____
_____
_____

Paradoxically, moving our bodies can help ease exhaustion by increasing our energy levels and boosting serotonin. At the same time, when we feel worn out, it's hard to get moving. What motivates you to be active? How can you fit more movement into your daily routine?

PLAN FOR REST

The weariness of grief can interfere with clear thinking, making it hard to recognize when we need to recuperate. Having go-to lists of indications that you need extra rest, what you need to recover, and whom you can call on for support takes some of the pressure off a weary mind. A sign of exhaustion might be losing your temper easily. You might need more sleep or someone to walk the dog this week. Include on your list the names of trusted friends, family members, and professionals (doctor, psychotherapist, etc.) on whom you can call for support and respite.

SIGNS I NEED REST	WAYS TO RECUPERATE	MY SUPPORT NETWORK

Exhaustion and the Need to Rest

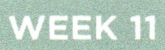

The Loneliness of Absence

I AM NOT ALONE IN MY GRIEF. I SHARE MY EXPERIENCE WITH EVERY PERSON WHO HAS LOST SOMEONE.

Grief makes us feel profoundly alone. Even others who share the loss can seem distant. At the same time, this loneliness is a common human experience. As you sit with the ways grief both disconnects and joins us, what kind words do you have for the lonely part of you?

I have often wished I could share some personal news with my father, something he alone would appreciate. Knowing I can't share these events with him is a lonely feeling. Are there things that have happened recently only your loved one would understand? Describe one thing you've wanted to share.

Being with others can help or it can deepen the pain. When we need contact but hanging out with friends or family is overwhelming, going to a public space, such as a park, helps. How do you know when you need to be with others? What public spaces feel comfortable to you?

Socializing takes energy that we don't always have. At the same time, spending time with family and friends can be healing. We can always take things slowly and leave early if we need to. Consider what you need right now. Whom could you spend time with? What are the signs you've had enough social time?

_____
_____
_____
_____
_____
_____
_____
_____

CONNECT WITH YOURSELF

Touch is powerful. By compassionately giving yourself a hug in front of a mirror, you can feel less alone. Sit or stand in front of a mirror, relaxing your shoulders as you take a few slow, deep breaths. Look at your reflection, maintaining eye contact, letting feelings of compassion and love expand in your body. Hug yourself by crossing your right arm over your chest and placing your hand near your heart. Then place your left hand on your right shoulder. Relax into the hug, allowing your feelings to flow through you. Stay with this position for as long as you want. What thoughts and feelings arise for you in this exercise?

WEEK 12

Feeling Abandoned

I AM NOT ALONE IN MY GRIEF. MY LOVED ONE LIVES WITHIN ME, A LOVE THAT NEVER DIES.

After someone dies, life seems empty. Our loved ones have gone missing. Familiar places become cavernous in their absence. We have been abandoned, left alone to wrestle with grief and its challenges. Give a voice to your feelings of abandonment. Are they angry or afraid? Devastated? Sad? All these and more? What might soothe these feelings?

Sometimes our feelings of abandonment after a death are familiar in their pain. Parents who deserted us, partners who disappeared without warning, or a childhood where we were left alone to process overwhelming emotions contribute to our current devastation. For some, those we mourn abandoned us well before dying. How do your previous experiences with abandonment affect your grief?

Though physically gone, our loved ones leave us emotional legacies. These legacies can be affirming, such as a sense of self-confidence or the knowledge we are lovable. They can come with baggage, such as feelings of rejection or mountains of debt. Affirming legacies often help us feel connected to our dead. Baggage-laden inheritances increase our feelings of abandonment. What emotional legacies did your loved one leave you?

Our loved ones are everywhere, and they are nowhere. Sometimes we feel them with us. They linger in the garden or occupy a seat at the breakfast table. They hover behind us as we load the dishwasher. There are places we visit to feel close to them. Where do you feel closest to your loved one?

DRAW YOUR TREE OF LIFE

Drawing a tree of life is a visual way to remind yourself of your strengths, your connections to the world and others, and what keeps you rooted. Begin from the roots up, using the following guide. Come back to your tree of life when you feel abandoned and unsettled.

Roots: Where you come from, early influences, family

Ground: Present-day activities you enjoy

Trunk: Your skills, values, and traits

Branches: Your hopes, dreams, and goals

Leaves: Important people in your life, including those who have passed away

Fruits: Gifts or legacies you've received from others

WEEK 13

Acknowledging Despair

I HOLD LIGHT WITHIN ME AND CAN SHINE THIS LIGHT THROUGH THE DARKNESS OF DESPAIR.

Feeling despair and hopelessness most of the day, nearly every day, for two weeks or more is a symptom of depression and a reason to talk to a psychotherapist or psychiatrist. If our despairing moods are sporadic and less persistent after loss, grief is likely behind our hopelessness. Describe your feelings of despair. Are they sporadic or more persistent? How often do you feel this way?

Despair can be a shield against heartbreak. With no hopes to dash, we feel safe from the pangs of unfulfilled yearning. The pain of no hope is better than the potential for hope to be destroyed. We end up stuck in the darkness, afraid of what it might mean to turn on a light. Does despair sometimes protect you against heartbreak? If so, how?

Grief has extinguished the spark within us. We lack energy and motivation. Despair tells us our inner light and sense of purpose are on permanent hiatus. Creating short- and long-term goals can keep us going in times of despair. What are some things you'd like to do over the next year? If identifying what you'd like to do is difficult, write out what needs to get done.

Acknowledging Despair

With our loved ones gone, it seems we can't go on. There is no point. But we do go on. Something within us fights against despair. Perhaps that something is love—for our dead, for our communities, for ourselves. Maybe we are motivated by ambition or some other desire tied to life. What within you keeps you going?

COMBAT DESPAIR

Small spontaneous, bright moments in life contradict despair's bleak outlook. For me, these might include petting a neighbor's cat or crunching autumn leaves under my feet. You can intentionally cultivate these moments of hope. Buying a flower bouquet, watching a funny movie, and relishing a good meal are all potential ways to create joy despite despair. Think about your happy, spontaneous moments. Consider ways to create these moments. Write them down as reminders of ways to combat despair.

HAPPY, SPONTANEOUS MOMENTS

HAPPY MOMENTS I CAN CREATE

WEEK 14

Coming to Terms with Changing Responsibilities

ALTHOUGH OTHERS DEPEND ON ME, MY NEEDS ARE ALSO IMPORTANT. I CREATE SPACE FOR MYSELF AND, AT THE SAME TIME, TAKE CARE OF MY RESPONSIBILITIES.

The death of someone important often affects our responsibilities. Sometimes we take on new tasks. Other times the list of things we attend to becomes shorter. Often it is only after a loss that we understand how many obligations our loved one carried. How has your loss changed your responsibilities?

In many families and friend groups, different people take on different tasks. For example, one person may host holiday gatherings, but another keeps track of birthdays or takes care of children. After a death, these responsibilities may be absorbed by others. Sometimes no one picks them up, and they simply stop happening. How has loss shifted responsibilities in your family or community?

Our loved ones are gone. We can no longer visit or attend to them. There is no "home" to return to or tasks to assist with. Their health or self-care has ceased to be a point of focus. The end of these responsibilities brings up various thoughts and feelings. What does it bring up for you?

Loss creates clarity. We carry the knowledge that life is finite and short. This clarity provides perspective, allowing us to approach our responsibilities with new appreciation or, if we are able, change what no longer serves us. In what ways has grief changed how you approach your responsibilities?

RECOGNIZING NEW PRIORITIES

Grief can take all the joy out of responsibilities you once enjoyed. Making meals becomes meaningless, and child-rearing a struggle. Perhaps your beloved job now feels like a slog. Sometimes these feelings are a temporary reaction to loss. Sometimes loss rearranges our priorities. It can take time to determine the difference. Write down two lists: one with your values and priorities prior to your loss, the other with your values and priorities as you see them now. How different are the lists? If they are different, what does this mean for how you want to prioritize responsibilities going forward?

VALUES BEFORE MY LOSS

Keeping the peace in my family

Work as a top priority

VALUES TODAY

Enforcing my boundaries

Maintaining relationships

WEEK 15

Choosing Rituals and Practices to Mark Your Loss

I USE RITUAL TO CONNECT TO MY LOVED ONE AND KEEP THEIR MEMORY ALIVE.

Many of us grow up absorbing religious or cultural practices around death and grief. These practices shape our beliefs about the "right" way to mark loss. They affect how we grieve and what we expect from others after a death. What rituals and practices around death and bereavement did you grow up with? How do they affect your grieving process today?

Sometimes we are expected to participate in grieving rituals that feel inauthentic to us or to the people we've lost. For example, we may be uncomfortable with certain funeral ceremonies or interment practices. Have you participated in rituals around your loss that felt uncomfortable to you? What about them was difficult?

_____
_____
_____
_____
_____
_____

Rituals connect us to the dead. These rituals can be religious, such as a funeral mass, or informal, such as pouring our loved one a drink graveside. Some rituals are annual. Others might be daily or happen once. What rituals do you use to honor and remember your loved one?

_____
_____
_____
_____
_____
_____

We aren't always able to recognize a loss through ritual, or the rituals we have participated in weren't helpful. Creating our own observances to mark our loss can help us process our feelings. What ritual could you create to honor your loved one and your relationship with them?

MAKE A SPACE FOR REMEMBRANCE

Gather items to create an altar or memorial for your loved one. This memorial can be as large or small as you would like it to be. Include things that you associate with the person you have lost, including photos, recordings, small objects, stones, crystals, scents, or important books and religious texts. A vase for fresh flowers and a bowl for offerings provide space for liveliness and devotion. Candles, votives, or small lamps add light. If you have an urn or some of your loved one's ashes, you can incorporate them into the altar. Decide if you want this memorial to be in a public or private place in your home, identifying an easy way to cover it if you wish.

WEEK 16

Handling Other Peoples' Expectations

I KNOW MYSELF BEST. I CHOOSE TO TAKE ADVICE THAT SERVES ME AND DISREGARD ADVICE THAT DOES NOT.

After a loss, we may receive suggestions on how to grieve. For example, a friend may tell us to start dating again, or a family member may advise us to give away our loved one's possessions. This advice is often well meaning, but it can also be painful. What unwanted advice about grief have you received? What feelings came up for you when you received it?

Some people may avoid us after a loss. Perhaps we remind them of the temporary nature of life or their own unprocessed grief. Their avoidance hurts. Give your wounded self a voice. What does it want to say to those made uncomfortable by your grief?

_____

_____

_____

_____

_____

_____

Other people's expectations and assumptions about the grieving process sometimes affect what we expect of ourselves. Even when these expectations don't quite fit, we may still try to meet them. For example, encouraged by well-meaning friends, we may put reminders of our loved one away against our wishes. How have you internalized others' expectations about grief? Do these expectations fit your needs? How or how not?

_____

_____

_____

_____

_____

_____

Handling Other Peoples' Expectations

Although some advice doesn't fit our needs, other guidance can be supportive and helpful. Folks who've been through loss or who know us well can provide us with both a helpful ear and wise counsel. What advice have you appreciated in your grief?

_____
_____
_____
_____
_____
_____
_____
_____

PRACTICE CREATING BOUNDARIES

Have your boundaries been stretched after your loss? Thinking through responses to unwanted advice in advance keeps your boundaries clear. Responses that are assertive, kind, and matter-of-fact convey your limits in a non-blaming way. Begin with an acknowledgment of the person's concern, and use "I" statements to soothe potential defensiveness. For example, if someone is pressuring you to date again, you could say, "I understand that you are concerned about me. However, I do not want to discuss my romantic life." Fill out the following potential responses.

I understand that you _____. However, I _____.

I recognize that you _____, but I _____.

I appreciate that you _____. For me, it is important I _____.

WEEK 17

Finding Meaning Through Tears

I ALLOW MYSELF TO CRY. MY TEARS ARE A TESTAMENT TO MY LOVE.

We absorb messages about crying from our families and cultures. These messages are often gendered. Crying is associated with weakness and femininity, but men and boys are taught to be "strong" and hold back tears. What beliefs do you hold about tears and crying? How do they affect your expressions of grief?

When you need to cry but can't, turning to sad movies, soulful music, or sentimental commercials can coax out tears. Video or audio recordings of your loved one, if you are ready for them, are another path to a cleansing cry. What do you turn to when you need to cry?

There are times in grief when the crying seems constant. I have dabbed away tears in work bathrooms, during meetings, at dinner, and while walking the dogs. Grief's watery intensity lessens, though significant dates and other reminders start the tap running again. Since your loss, when have tears overwhelmed you?

Tears can be an offering to our loved one, an acknowledgment of their importance. They can express our absolute devastation in loss or come from anger and overwhelm. Tell the story of your tears.

VISUALIZE TEARS AS RAIN

Sit in a comfortable position. Close your eyes if you wish. Take a few slow, deep breaths. You are back as your tree of life from Week 12, deeply rooted and connected to your fellow trees. It has been a long dry spell. The ground is dusty. Your roots are thirsty, and your limbs droop in the afternoon sun. A slight breeze picks up as the sky clouds over. The air becomes heavy with humidity, and light rain starts to fall. Drops slide off your leaves and branches and sink into the ground. The rain picks up, making a pattering sound on your branches. Your roots drink up the moisture. Your limbs perk up. Slowly, the rain stops. The sun emerges, making glints of the drops on your leaves. You are calm and satiated. Open your eyes when you are ready.

[Record yourself reading this exercise, speaking slowly. Play it back to begin the visualization.]

WEEK 18

Facing Reminders

I ALLOW MYSELF TO FEEL WHATEVER COMES UP WHEN REMINDED OF MY LOSS. I SAVOR HAPPY FEELINGS AND KNOW DIFFICULT ONES WILL PASS.

Reminders of our loved ones and their deaths can be painful. It is natural to want to avoid them in hopes of escaping deep sadness. However, this avoidance can prevent us from processing our feelings. Rather than decreasing the ache of loss, avoidance extends it. What reminders are you avoiding?

We know the people we grieve are not coming back. But sometimes encountering reminders of all we have lost sharpens that knowledge, intensifying our pain. These reminders may bring up other difficult feelings such as guilt, anger, or fear. What feelings arise when you are reminded of your loved one?

Many reminders can be anticipated. Familiar places, old routines, or a loved one's favorite foods can all bring them vividly to mind. But reminders also take us by surprise. Perhaps we hear a favorite song when out shopping, or come across an unexpected photo memory. Write about a time when you were reminded of your loved one out of the blue.

Some reminders help us recall joyful moments. My grandmother's recipe box not only brings her to mind, but it also brings back the (bad!) cooking of my childhood. It makes me smile. What positive reminders do you have of your loved ones? If there are no positive reminders, what might become positive over time?

PLAN FOR REMINDERS

When reminders intensify grief, having a plan for acknowledging and processing your feelings can help you tolerate them. This plan should include ways to sit with and work through your emotions by, for example, writing out your thoughts and feelings in a notebook, lighting a candle or incense, or meditating. Self-care activities, like taking a bath, watching sad or funny movies, listening to music, or eating a soothing and nutritious meal should also be on your list. If possible, include at least one person you can call on who understands what you are going through.

WEEK 19

Feeling Like No One Understands

**I FIND STRENGTH AND DEEP UNDERSTANDING
IN MYSELF AS I GRIEVE.**

People tell us they know how we feel after our loss. They make assumptions about our emotional state and suggestions for coping. We nod without comment or mutter thanks, but inside we seethe and ache. What would you like people to understand about your grief?

It is painful to be misunderstood in our grief. We feel apart from others, strange, somehow wrong. Sometimes these feelings echo experiences in our pasts, other times when we've felt like the odd person out. This misunderstood part of us deserves compassion. What kind words do you have for the part of you no one gets?

_____
_____
_____
_____
_____
_____

If no one knows how we feel, we also may not know how they feel. Feeling compassion and letting go of our assumptions about the intentions of others is freeing. They may be dealing with their own hidden grief or complicated loss. How can you cultivate compassion toward the clueless?

_____
_____
_____
_____
_____
_____
_____

Our grief separates us from friends and family. Though we are alone in it, clinging to our separateness becomes a barrier to connection and healing. Feelings of alienation keep us alienated. Have you put up walls between yourself and others? When do they protect you? When do they isolate you?

VISUALIZE CONNECTION

Sit in a comfortable position. Close your eyes if you wish. Take a few slow, deep breaths. Imagine yourself as the tree of life (Week 12). Your roots go deep into the ground. Your branches reach up into the sky. You are healthy and full, thick with leaves and fruit. You grow in a forest of other trees—some of them are like you, and some are completely different. Under the ground, your roots intermingle with the others. Across the canopy, your branches touch those of your neighbors. You share the air and sky, drink in the same rain, are battered by storms and wind together. Take solace in what you share with your fellow trees. They experience your pain and joy. You feel deeply connected and understood in this forest. When you are ready, open your eyes.

> Record yourself reading this exercise, speaking slowly. Play it back to begin the visualization.

WEEK 20

The Burden of Regret

I RELEASE ANY REGRET I CARRY AROUND MY LOVED ONE AND OFFER MYSELF COMPASSION AND FORGIVENESS.

After someone is gone, we can get stuck in our regret, caught up in the things we wish we had never said or done. Our harsh words or cruel actions haunt us, and our thoughts trap us in a loop of guilt. Writing out our regrets makes them more manageable. What are your regrets around your loved one?

Our emotions are expressed in our bodies. For example, we may feel anxiety in our stomachs or find that words get caught in our throats when we are nervous. Sit for a moment with your feelings of regret, taking a few slow, deep breaths as you check in. Where does regret show up in your body? What is it like to notice it?

> **If checking in with your body is overwhelming, stop and ground yourself by using your senses, noting the things you can see, smell, touch, and hear around you.**

Death removes all opportunity to make amends directly to our loved ones. There are no more chances to apologize or talk about how we feel or what we would do differently. What would you like your loved one to know about the things you regret?

The Burden of Regret

We cannot change the past, but we can take the lessons we learn from our regret into the future. As we make different choices, we can let go of regret and feel compassion toward ourselves. What have you learned from your regrets?

_____
_____
_____
_____
_____
_____
_____
_____
_____
_____

WRITE A GOODBYE NOTE TO REGRET

Writing a goodbye note to your regret allows you to acknowledge the role it has played in your grief. Use the note to tell regret what it has taught you and how you will integrate its lessons going forward. For example, if you regret something you said to your loved one, you might thank regret for reminding you of the importance of thinking before you speak, and then note how you are now more careful choosing your words. End with a warm goodbye.

WEEK 21

Finding Yourself Again

**AS I PROCESS MY GRIEF, I UNCOVER AND
REDISCOVER PARTS OF MYSELF. I HAVE
FAITH I WILL FEEL WHOLE AGAIN.**

Often it is only after someone is gone that we understand how our identities were interwoven with theirs. Who are we in their absence? We grieve not only our loved ones but also what we've lost of ourselves. What parts of your identity were tied to your loved one? Describe how your sense of self has changed since your loss.

Our lives and selves are broken into pieces, fractured by grief. We don't feel strong at the broken places, just shattered and in shards. Naming our feelings and fears supports healing and wholeness. Writing them down makes them feel real but also more manageable. What has grief broken in you?

What was once familiar about us feels foreign and distant. Grief muddies our sense of who we are. You are a grieving person. You may also be a friend, a dancer, or an administrative assistant, but the role of griever sometimes takes over. Are there roles on hold for you right now? What are they?

Grief and mourning are sticky, stuck places. We don't want to change because changing feels like an abandonment of those we have lost. The process of change sounds exhausting anyway. But we are here, alive. Change is still possible. What does it mean to hold out the hope for self-discovery?

REENGAGE WITH YOURSELF

After a loss, we may reengage with these long-forgotten pieces of ourselves, some going back to our early days. Think back to an activity you enjoyed as a child. It could be anything, such as reading, drawing, playing sports, or enjoying flights of the imagination. Close your eyes and imagine yourself back in time, deeply involved in this joyful activity. Occupy this early version of yourself, paying attention to your surroundings, and noticing the sensations and feelings that emerge. Open your eyes when you are ready. What of this past activity would you like to incorporate into your life today?

WEEK 22

Sitting with Unresolved, Prolonged, or Complicated Grief

THOUGH MY FEELINGS ABOUT MY LOSS ARE DIFFICULT TO BEAR, I AM STRONG AND CAN WEATHER THIS GRIEF.

Some losses are difficult to make sense of. Sudden deaths or ones we were not present for are often particularly hard to mourn. Ambiguous losses of loved ones, to degenerative or mental illnesses or unclear circumstances, are also hard to process. What, if any, of your loss is unresolved, ambiguous, or complicated?

_____
_____
_____
_____
_____
_____
_____

The death of someone with whom we had a difficult relationship can lead to complicated feelings around their loss. Sometimes death creates space for us to view them with compassion. It may leave us relieved. Sometimes we feel cheated or angry. How does the relationship you had with your loved one affect your grief?

When a loved one's death was painful or full of suffering, letting go of guilt is hard. We may obsess over what we could have done differently or worry about their final moments. These thinking patterns are hard to break. What images, thoughts, and feelings around your loved one's death would you like to release?

It may seem that our grief will never feel tolerable. Though we can recognize its complications and ambiguities, the idea that we will move through it or feel differently is hard to imagine. What are your hopes for handling the ambiguities and complications of your grief?

_____
_____
_____
_____
_____
_____
_____
_____

HOLD TWO TRUTHS

Ambiguous loss occurs when a loved one is physically or psychologically absent. Examples include grieving someone who is missing, has dementia, or is incarcerated. Psychologist Pauline Boss, an expert in ambiguous loss, recommends cultivating flexibility in your grief by holding two seemingly opposite truths about your loss simultaneously. For example, if you have a partner with dementia, you might say, "My partner is alive, and the partner I remember is gone." If your father has been imprisoned most of your life, you might think, "I have a father, and I do not have a father." Spend a few minutes thinking two truths you hold, either in your grief or in other situations.

WEEK 23

Making Decisions, Big and Little

I DON'T HAVE TO MAKE ANY DECISIONS TODAY. I ALLOW MYSELF SPACE AND TIME TO THINK ABOUT WHAT I NEED AND WANT.

Loss rearranges our relationships, adds and subtracts responsibilities, and creates situations in which we must make decisions. These decisions can be existential, focused on how we choose to live the rest of our lives. They can be practical, such as deciding to downsize. What decisions has loss presented to you?

We have a variety of feelings about the decisions we must make after loss. Overwhelm, confusion, and excitement are all normal responses. Perhaps your loss has given you the freedom to make changes. Maybe it has forced you to make uncomfortable or unwelcome choices. What feelings arise around the decisions you've made because of your loss?

When grief is all-encompassing, it can be difficult to make necessary decisions. We may put off these decisions because making them means making changes, and making changes pulls us away from those we've lost. Are there decisions you have been putting off? What gets in the way?

Sometimes we rush to make big decisions shortly after a loss, perhaps circumventing grief through distraction or avoidance. Immediately giving away our loved one's things or moving away may sound appealing, but it is best to wait until you've had some time to process your loss to make these decisions. Have you made big decisions since your loss? What motivated these decisions?

___

MAKE DECISIONS MINDFULLY

When decisions present themselves after loss, thinking through your motivations and needs helps you make mindful choices. Use this template to structure your thought process as you consider the decisions awaiting you.

Decision I May Need to Make: ___

Motivation for This Decision: ___

My Options: ___

Potential Consequences of Making This Decision: ___

Potential Consequences of Not Making This Decision: ___

WEEK 24

Am I Grieving, Depressed, or Both?

I PAY ATTENTION TO HOW I FEEL AND GET SUPPORT IF THE INTENSE SADNESS OF MY GRIEF DEEPENS INTO DEPRESSION.

If we have a family history of depression, have been depressed in the past, or have experienced trauma, we are more at risk for developing depression after loss. Identifying our vulnerabilities helps us focus proactively on emerging symptoms, self-care, and support. What, if any, risk factors for depression do you have?

The magnitude of grief can be confused with depression. Our obvious, deep sadness sometimes leads concerned or uncomfortable friends and family to suggest our bereavement is abnormal or that we need help.

Our capacity to process grief depends in part on what we've learned about coping with loss. If our families or cultures discourage directly expressing sadness around loss, we may find ourselves struggling now. Without an outlet, grief can turn into depression. How did the people you grew up with talk, or not talk, about death, loss, and grief?

Many things influence how we think and feel about depression, from our experiences with mental illness to the stigmas around it. This can make it tricky to identify in ourselves. In my case, watching my father's lifelong struggle with treatment-resistant depression affected how I interpreted my own symptoms. I spent years without treatment. With acceptance of my symptoms, psychotherapy, and medication eventually brought relief. What are your beliefs or experiences around depression or other mental health challenges? How might those beliefs affect how you interpret potential symptoms? Cultivate gentleness toward yourself as you navigate these difficult feelings.

CHECK YOUR SYMPTOMS

Mark off the symptoms you are experiencing in the following chart, including their frequency. If you've experienced a few of these most of the day nearly every day for two weeks or more, you may be depressed and should seek support from a psychotherapist. Check the Resources section at the back of the book for ways to find professional support. If you are feeling actively suicidal, call the National Suicide Prevention Lifeline at 1-800-273-8255.

SYMPTOM	LESS THAN HALF THE TIME	MORE DAYS THAN NOT	NEARLY ALL THE TIME
Little to no appetite or overeating			
Sleeping too much or having trouble sleeping			
Feeling sad			
Difficulty concentrating/focusing			
Fatigue and loss of energy			
Feeling worthless, guilty, or like a failure			
Feeling hopeless			
Thoughts of suicide or a wish to be dead			

Am I Grieving, Depressed, or Both?

WEEK 25

Acknowledging Stuck Points

WHEN I FEEL STUCK, I AM PATIENT WITH MYSELF. THE FEELING IS TEMPORARY AND MEANS I HAVE EMOTIONS TO PROCESS.

After a loss, we may feel trapped by circumstances out of our control. Our paths are blocked, our choices limited. It is true that grief sometimes puts us into unwelcome situations. We can quickly feel stuck. Where have you felt stuck since losing your loved one?

_____

_____

_____

_____

_____

_____

_____

_____

_____

_____

Not only can we feel stuck in circumstance, but we also can get caught up in ways of thinking and feeling. Some emotions or beliefs are hard to let go of, particularly when paired with the ache of loss. What feelings or beliefs tied to your loss would you like to release?

There are times when we are tired of grief. We wonder if the sadness will ever lessen. We feel stuck and frustrated. This is an understandable reaction to the slog of grief. Cultivating acceptance and being kind to ourselves helps us feel less stuck. Write some encouraging words to help you weather grief's relentlessness.

Imagining ourselves becoming unstuck opens room for change and clarifies our needs. Consider your stuck places in grief, situations currently out of your control, or hard-to-shake feelings and thoughts tied to your loss. If you could be instantly freed from these stuck points, what might change for you?

COPE THROUGH RADICAL ACCEPTANCE

Radical acceptance is a therapeutic technique that helps you cope with the frustration and pain of feeling stuck. Anger at what is out of your control can block you from seeing and accepting reality. When you see things realistically, your frustration can lessen. Opportunities for change may emerge as you gain clarity through acceptance. To use radical acceptance, first pay attention to your resistance to situations you cannot change. Remind yourself that there are reasons things are this way. When this gets overwhelming, calm yourself through 4-7-8 breathing (Week 7), butterfly tapping (Week 45), or meditative drawing (Week 31). How would you feel and act if you accepted reality? How would you feel if you continued to fight against it? Acknowledge and sit with the feelings that arise with radical acceptance.

WEEK 26

Mourning Intimacy and Connection

**WHEN MISSING MY LOVED ONE FEELS UNBEARABLE,
I REMIND MYSELF THAT MY PAIN IS TIED TO LOVE.**

Intimacy takes many forms, from the emotional to the physical. It can include sex, yes, but also cuddling or back massages or a knowing glance across a crowded room. Intimacy is linked to trust, a shared history, to being known and loved despite our flaws. What aspects of intimacy with your loved one do you miss?

There are things that only our lost loved ones would understand, jokes only they would get, secrets only they would keep. These tidbits seem less real without a person to share them with. They fade away. What would you like to share with your loved one that they alone would understand?

When a person dies, the intimacy we shared also dies. We know them deeply, from personality to physicality. But they are gone, and we remain here, bereft. Our missing takes the form of an ache. Some days are worse than others. When do you most miss the presence of your loved one?

Whether our loved one was a friend, partner, or relative, intimate relationships are daunting after loss. We may fear that having new intimate relationships shows disloyalty to our loved ones. An intimate relationship may feel completely off the table, forever. Or perhaps we are lonely and ready to connect. How do you feel about starting an intimate relationship after your loss?

_____
_____
_____
_____
_____
_____
_____
_____

CREATE A TOUCH KIT

In the aftermath of death, touch can become elusive or overwhelming, a reminder of the person and the physical contact you miss. Put together a kit for incorporating more touch into your life. Choose a few small items with pleasing textures such as fleece, cotton balls, a pliable squishy, or putty. Add a sleeping bag or a weighted blanket for those times you need to be wrapped up tight and a body pillow when you want to cuddle close. If possible, add activities to your kit, including time with people or pets (yours or someone else's) and bubble baths or massages.

What will you include in your kit?

WEEK 27

Your Feelings About Changing Relationships

I DESERVE LOVE AND KINDNESS. I WELCOME NEW FRIENDSHIPS AND LET GO OF UNHEALTHY ONES.

Death can rearrange and prune relationships. Close friends disappear or spout clueless advice. Acquaintances become trusted companions. Family members vary in their ability to be present. Being abandoned or treated carelessly in our time of need hurts. How has loss changed and challenged your relationships?

New friends nourish us, giving us hope for the future and a fresh audience for stories about our loved ones. But new friendships are also bittersweet. Our friends will never meet the people we've lost, and our loved ones will never meet them. What feelings arise when you think about forming new friendships?

After a loss, what we seek out of friendship can change. Consider the characteristics you love in your friends and family or ones you wish they had. Combine these positive attributes to make a virtual super friend. What qualities are you looking for?

Forming relationships post-loss is anxiety-provoking. We worry about being hurt or rejected, which leads us to conceal our tender or less appealing qualities. Or perhaps we are eager to explore new connections, open and excited about experiencing something new. When approaching new friendships after loss, what have you revealed? What have you concealed?

CONNECT PAST, PRESENT, AND FUTURE RELATIONSHIPS

Make a collage linking your present and past relationships, choosing materials that represent your relationships before your loss, how they stand now, and how you would like them to be. Use photographs, letters, email, or materials cut out of magazines and books that symbolize or reflect your feelings around friendships. Include construction paper, tissue paper, or other objects to add color and texture, along with something sturdy, like a piece of cardboard, to affix them to. Depending on how you feel and what you want the collage to represent, carefully cut the items out, rip them apart, or do both. Be deliberate about how you juxtapose the pieces, arranging them in a meaningful way. What title fits your collage?

WEEK 28

Honoring Your Loved One

I HONOR MY LOVED ONE BY LIVING MY LIFE FULLY AND KEEPING THEIR MEMORY ALIVE.

We honor our loved ones in both public and private ways. For example, donating to charity in their names or dedicating park benches to their memory shares them with others directly. Choosing to be kind or generous in their honor is a private homage. In what ways do you honor your loved one?

Wakes, funerals, and memorial services are ceremonial events honoring our loved ones. Although these events center around loss, they also celebrate life. Sometimes we have input into planning these celebrations. Sometimes we don't. If it were completely up to you, how would you honor your loved one in a joyful event?

Sometimes grief takes away our intrinsic motivation to stay engaged in life. We lose our desire to take care of ourselves or connect to others. But reinvesting in our lives is a way of honoring our dead. What do you do for yourself in honor of your loved one?

Writing an obituary allows us to record our loved ones' life stories. It also lets other people know how our loved ones lived and that they have died. Some obituaries include personal details, but most leave out the personal and list significant achievements. What would you include in an obituary honoring your loved one's personal qualities?

CREATE A MEMORY BOX

Choose something to use as a box. This can be anything from a shoebox to a wooden crate. Decorate the box with paint or special paper, a photo of your loved one, or anything that represents and honors them. If you aren't crafty, or if a plain box is a better fit, feel free to skip this step. Gather items connected to your loved one to put in your memory box. These can include photographs; copies of notes, emails, letters, or texts; significant objects, such as jewelry or books; and anything related to their interests or your relationship. Include your own letter describing the ways you intend to honor your loved one's memories, using this week's prompts for inspiration.

WEEK 29

Accepting the Passage of Time

I AM ALIVE NOW. I CHOOSE TO LIVE IN THE PRESENT AND CAN IMAGINE A HOPEFUL FUTURE.

Moving forward in time leaves our lost loved ones behind. Living in the past keeps us stuck. We become trapped and stagnant, worried that changing and growing mean being disloyal to the dead. How would your loved one feel about your becoming reengaged in life? How might they encourage you to live in the present?

_____

_____

_____

_____

_____

_____

_____

_____

_____

_____

_____

_____

After a loss, it is normal to fantasize about turning back the clock. Being with our loved ones again and saving them from their fates are common themes. These fantasies bring comfort. They sometimes bring pain. What would you do if you could time travel back to your loved one?

_____
_____
_____
_____
_____

The platitude "time heals all wounds" does not apply to grief. Our wounds become a part of us, tender marks on the psyche, reminders of whom and what we've lost. However, our relationship with these wounds can change over time. How do your wounds feel now? How do you hope they will feel in a year?

_____
_____
_____
_____
_____
_____

Grief freezes our lives at the moment of loss. Still, life unfurls before us. We may want to plan for the future but are caught in the past. Or we find a future without our loved ones too painful to contemplate. What are your feelings about the future?

ANTICIPATE THE FUTURE

Loss divides life into before and after. Before can be a joyful yet rough place to visit, a museum of memory. The time after a loss is bleak, filled with the dread of dates and the fresh pain they bring. This timeline invites you to anticipate the future, however you want to define it, but at the same time note significant events in the past. As you consider the future, mark dates related to your loss, such as birthdays and anniversaries. If you can, include a few things you look forward to. Upcoming milestones, planned events, and hopeful goals can intermingle with the more difficult dates, a sign that loss and life can coexist.

BEFORE   **LOSS**   **AFTER**

Accepting the Passage of Time

WEEK 30

Finding Your People

I SHARE MY EXPERIENCES WITH OTHERS AND RECEIVE STRENGTH AND SUPPORT FROM MY COMMUNITIES.

We feel alone. We want to be alone. But can we get through grief alone? Some of us are introverts, used to holding our own counsel, wary of crowds. Other are extroverts who feel best in the middle of a pack. No matter our orientation, having support from folks who have also experienced loss helps. How do you feel about joining grief support groups?

Sometimes after a loss, our communities dissipate and change. People we once counted on for emotional support vanish or construct barricades to connection. Other times our communities rally around us, helping us feel less alone. What has happened to your communities in the wake of your grief?

Creating or joining a community after experiencing a death is an investment in ourselves. It provides a fresh focus, allowing us to reengage with life. At the same time, it is daunting to set out on a new course with new people. It can also feel like an abandonment of our loved one. Perhaps it feels impossible or unappealing to start afresh. What are your feelings, fears, and hopes around finding community?

Participating in a community by volunteering or contributing our time connects us to others. It is also good for our mental health, as long as we're careful not to overextend ourselves. Are there ways you contribute to a community? How? Why?

___

IDENTIFY YOUR COMMUNITIES

Even when it seems there is no place you belong, you are connected to communities. Draw four concentric circles on a blank sheet of paper, allowing room to write within each. Put your name in the center circle. In the next circle, write the names of family and close friends, including those who have passed away. The third circle is for acquaintances, people you interact with casually, such as coworkers or neighbors. The final circle should include those who provide support and services, such as the mail deliverer, your psychotherapist, health care workers, or the waitstaff at your favorite restaurant. Add circles for other communities you participate in.

WEEK 31

Transcending Loss Through Creativity, Art, and Music

**ART CONNECTS ME TO JOY, SADNESS, AND MEMORIES.
I CHOOSE TO BRING MORE ART INTO MY LIFE.**

We transcend grief and experience moments of relief by connecting to something bigger than ourselves. One way to do this is by getting lost in a painting or photograph. Another could be to attend a concert or religious ceremony. Some of us write poetry or choreograph dance. How do you use art to transcend your grief?

Anthems are songs written in praise and celebration of nations, groups of people, or cultures. Examples include Lady Gaga's "Born This Way," an anthem for the LGBTQIA+ community, and the hymn "Lift Every Voice and Sing," an anthem for the civil rights movement. What would you title an anthem to you and your loved one? Why?

_____
_____
_____
_____
_____

Art taps into emotion, allowing us to cry or connect with feelings we didn't know we had. It could be a painting that breaks our hearts open or perhaps a dance piece. Maybe we are profoundly touched by a poem. What artworks or performances have been meaningful to you in your grief?

_____
_____
_____
_____
_____
_____

Music is a full-bodied experience. Some songs make us shimmy and shout, coaxing our bodies briefly out of sadness. Other songs vibrate into our core, tapping into the bone-deep ache of our grief. The intensity may be welcome, or it may overwhelm us. How have you been affected by music since your loss?

CALM YOUR FEELINGS THROUGH MEDITATIVE DRAWING

When you are struggling and overwhelmed by loss, meditative drawing can calm your mind, emotions, and body. By focusing completely on the act of creating, you can feel more centered and relaxed. This activity also directs your attention away from the feelings of despair and disconnection that come with grief. No drawing experience or abilities are necessary. To begin, grab a pencil or pen and a sheet of paper, and sit comfortably with a relaxed hand. Fill the page with hatch marks arranged in a pattern. Build a larger drawing out of interconnected squiggles. Draw a series of circles that build on each other. Create a spiral and fill in the space between the lines with patterns. Or simply put pencil to paper or stylus to screen and enjoy the sensation of making a connection with a surface. If drawing is difficult for you, enlist a friend or family member to guide or support your hand. The only requirement is to let your hand and mind freely relax as you draw.

WEEK 32

Gathering Your Memories

MY LOVED ONE LIVES ON IN MY STORIES AND MEMORIES. WHAT WE SHARED TOGETHER CANNOT BE TAKEN AWAY.

Sometimes death makes us the sole caretaker of memories, the only one who remembers the inside jokes, tender moments, or tough times. This is a painful experience. Sharing these memories with others keeps them alive. Describe one memory you are the sole keeper of. Who could you share it with?

After a person is gone, we can be haunted by memories that make us feel angry, guilty, or full of regret. The past cannot be changed, but the importance that we give to these memories can be lessened over time. What memories do you hope will lose their sting?

My first visit to my father and stepmother's house after his death made his loss real all over again. Reminders of him were everywhere, and grief struck me anew. Are there places you avoid or constantly visit because you associate them with your loved one? How does being in these spaces affect you?

After a loss, recalling a funny shared memory is bittersweet. In the moment of remembering, the past comes to life. Happiness is followed by the ache of missing. Remember a time when you and your loved one laughed together. Record this memory in the space that follows and let your emotions be without judgment.

ASSOCIATE SCENTS WITH MEMORIES

The sense of smell is closely linked to memory. Catching a whiff of a familiar scent transports us to a different time and place. When someone dies, their scent becomes elusive, though particular fragrances can bring them vividly back to life. Choose an item whose scent reminds you of your loved one. A perfume or cologne, a food, and even a piece of clothing are examples. Set aside five to fifteen minutes to sit with this object. Take in its scent. Let your mind and heart wander, going where the fragrance leads them, closing your eyes if you wish. Images, memories, associations, and strong emotions may all surface. Stop at any time if you feel overwhelmed. If this exercise brings comfort, repeat with different scents.

WEEK 33

Keeping Connected to Your Loved One

I GIVE MYSELF PERMISSION TO DO HARMLESS THINGS THAT KEEP ME CONNECTED TO MY LOVED ONE.

We sometimes do unexpected or unusual things to keep us connected with our lost loved ones. Other people might judge us or think our actions are unwise, but we aren't hurting anyone, and our actions bring us comfort. What unusual things have you done in the name of grief?

It is common to keep reminders of loved ones long past their deaths or do things like continue to set a place for them at the table or speak to their photos. There may be other things that we'd like to do but are worried they might be perceived as strange, so we hold off. What have you wanted to do in your grief but have been afraid to?

Some objects remind us of our loved ones more than others. I still have a cap that belonged to my mother's partner, one he wore often and was photographed in. That cap has crossed the country with me, a tangible reminder of him. What one object reminds you most of your loved one? Why?

Sometimes we want to stop some of the things we do out of grief. But stopping can feel like forgetting or being disloyal to our loved ones. Or doing these things keeps us from processing our loved ones' deaths. We fear what will happen if we stop. As a griever, are there things you want to stop doing? What makes stopping hard?

_____
_____
_____
_____
_____
_____
_____
_____
_____
_____

LEAVE YOUR LOVED ONE A MESSAGE

Use the recording feature on your smartphone to leave your loved one a message. Say whatever you'd like. You can plan out your message or see what emerges when you hit record. Do you want to catch them up on the happenings in your life, remind them of your love, or yell at them for leaving? Perhaps you don't want to say anything but want to feel them there, listening to you. Or you want to say how much you miss them. If you don't have a smartphone, you can record your message using an audio recording device. You can also just speak into a phone without recording.

WEEK 34

Looking for Signs

I AM OPEN TO RECEIVING SIGNS FROM MY LOVED ONE AND TAKE THEM AS MESSAGES OF LOVE.

Some of us believe our loved ones can send us signs after death. Others think this is unlikely or impossible. Even when we don't believe in signs, we may find ourselves hoping for, or seeing them, despite ourselves. What are your beliefs about signs from the dead?

Signs from our loved ones could be extremely personal, something only we would understand. They could be more universally recognizable, such as a cardinal sighting on a significant date or coins showing up in unexpected places. Have you received signs from your loved one? What were they?

Some dreams about our loved ones feel like signs from beyond. They stick with us. Shortly after my husband's father died, I dreamed he raised a glass to me across a crowded restaurant. "I hope you have a wonderful life," he said, smiling. I haven't dreamed of him since. Have any of your dreams felt like visitations? Describe them.

It causes no harm to interpret potential coincidences or unlikely occurrences as signs from our dead. Even if they aren't direct communications, they are indications we remain connected to our loved ones and see evidence of our love in the world. What potential signs have you discounted?

INVITE AND ACCEPT SIGNS

Get into a comfortable seated position and take a few slow, deep breaths. Close your eyes if you wish. Empty your mind of any skepticism or doubt about signs from the beyond. Create a feeling of spaciousness within your mind, an openness to noticing and acknowledging communications from your loved one. If you have struggled with the veracity of signs, use this time to set aside doubt and accept past potential signs as evidence of the love you continue to share with the person you've lost. As your doubt melts away, invite your loved one to continue to connect with you through signs and dreams, cultivating openness and a feeling of connection. If your acceptance of signs continues to feel unlikely, use this meditation to encourage openness about signs as reminders of your loved one and what you shared. When you are done, slowly open your eyes.

WEEK 35

Anticipating Birthdays, Anniversaries, and Holidays

I OFFER MYSELF COMPASSION AND ALLOW ROOM FOR MY GRIEF ON IMPORTANT DATES AND CELEBRATIONS.

After a loss, the holiday joy of others often deepens our pain. It can feel inconceivable that anyone could be happy when our loved one is gone forever. We may despair of ever feeling joy around holidays again. What are your feelings or worries about celebrating holidays without your loved one?

We are prepared for grief to hit us on holidays, birthdays, or anniversaries and even on more personal significant dates. But there are also the events that our loved one will never experience, such as graduations, weddings, or births. These can bring grief up all over again in surprising ways. What feelings arise for you when considering these celebratory events? How will you get through them?

Special occasions can lose their appeal after a loss. They don't feel the same without our loved ones. We just go through the motions. Choosing to celebrate in different ways can help us get through those occasions, even if we choose to ignore them. How will you mark these occasions without your loved one?

Our loved ones will never be part of our celebrations again. It is easy to get lost in this painful fact. Still, some birthdays, holidays, and anniversaries are significant because of our love for and connection to our loved ones. Perhaps this love can help us stand the pain. How could you lean into your love to help you with your pain around significant dates?

_____

_____

_____

_____

_____

_____

_____

PREPARE FOR SIGNIFICANT DATES

People expect grievers to feel sad on the big dates, such as major holidays. But the invisible annual events, such as death or wedding anniversaries or other dates of personal significance, can go unnoticed. Anticipating these dates and your feelings around them, as well as what you will need to get through them, can help prepare you for hard times ahead. For example, on the anniversary of a loved one's diagnosis, you may feel sad and angry and will need time alone.

SIGNIFICANT DATE	HOW I WILL FEEL	WHAT I WILL NEED
_____	_____	_____
_____	_____	_____
_____	_____	_____

WEEK 36

Nurturing Hope

**IN MY GRIEF, I NURTURE MY HOPE AND
ALLOW IT TO GROW AND BLOOM.**

Sometimes we are not ready to feel hopeful. Our loved one has died, and we need time to sit with our grief. It is impossible to identify bright spots in our devastated world. Are you ready for hope? How do you feel about cultivating hope after your loss?

In some areas of grief, we may be hopeful, but in others we feel despair. Perhaps we hope we will date casually but despair over (or can't even think about) feeling connected to another person again. Where do you feel despair? Where do you feel hope?

Poet Emily Dickinson compared hope to a bird that sings despite the hardships of life ("Hope is the thing with feathers"). Hope is the light at the end of the tunnel. It is the sun peeking through clouds. For me, hope is a budding zinnia about to burst into bloom. How would you describe the hope you nurture in grief?

Bad things have happened to us. We've lost people we love. Though our loss overshadows the good things in life, it does not completely cancel them out. Identifying and accepting what remains good feeds hope and strengthens resilience. What are some good things in your life?

_____
_____
_____
_____
_____
_____
_____
_____

MAKE SPACE FOR HOPE

Sit in a comfortable position, taking a few slow, deep breaths. Close your eyes if you wish. Imagine a warm ball of light hovering above you. This light is soothing, safe, and reassuring. Allow the light to enter your body at the top of your head. It moves gently and slowly from your head to your neck, expanding throughout your torso before traveling to your arms, hands, and fingers, finally working its way to your legs, feet, and toes. As it moves, it melts away despair, filling you with possibility and hope. Sit with this feeling, noticing any other emotions and sensations that emerge without judgment. Stop at any time if you feel overwhelmed. You are safe. Emotions come and go. When you are done, slowly open your eyes.

WEEK 37

Recognizing Sudden Bouts of Grief

I AM PATIENT WITH MYSELF WHEN I AM OVERWHELMED BY GRIEF AND GIVE MYSELF TIME TO PROCESS MY FEELINGS.

Grief attacks seem to come out of nowhere. One moment we're fine, the next our heart rate is skyrocketing, and we're rushing out of the grocery store. Though these attacks and moods may catch us by surprise, there are probably precipitating events, or triggers, that set us off. What triggers your grief attacks?

Grief is a maelstrom of emotion inside us, a storm of epic proportions. It can take all our focus and energy. When the intensity is overwhelming, we go into survival mode. What do you do when your emotions feel like too much?

We can't avoid all triggers, but we can choose how we respond to them. For example, looking at my father's photos after his death was crushing, so I didn't. Eventually, I decided to see them as joyful artifacts of his life. Now they remind me of him in a loving, sometimes bittersweet way. What grief responses would you like to reframe?

Externalizing emotions helps us better understand and manage them. Identify an emotion you are challenged by in your grief. Imagine this emotion as a character, a part of you that you can observe, empathize with, and engage with. Give it a name and features. What emotion did you pick? What is its name? What does it look like?

_____

_____

_____

_____

_____

TAKE A MINDFUL APPROACH

Grief attacks knock us down. A mindful approach makes them tolerable. Practicing mindfulness in calmer moments makes it easier to use when you are overwhelmed.

1. **Check in with how you are feeling right now. Pay attention to the sensations in your body as well as your thoughts.**
2. **Name the emotion.**
3. **Remind yourself that the emotion is temporary, opening space to choose your response.**
4. **Choose how you respond to the emotion.**

> **For example:** *My shoulders are tense. My thoughts are racing. I'm nervous and can't concentrate. Ah, I'm feeling anxious. This anxiety will pass. I'm going to pay less attention to my racing thoughts and will try 4-7-8 breathing to calm myself.*

WEEK 38

What I Didn't Expect About Grief

I LEARN NEW THINGS ABOUT MYSELF AND OTHERS IN MY GRIEF AND CAN HANDLE THE UNEXPECTED.

There are things we may not have expected about bereavement. Sometimes our experience matches our expectations with few surprises. Other times we have had to discard all we thought we knew of the grieving process. What aspects of your grief have been unexpected?

_____

_____

_____

_____

_____

_____

_____

_____

_____

Many of us come to grief with misperceptions about how we will feel. Loss gives us new perspective. Our lived experience can soften and broaden our attitudes about grief, deepening empathy for others or past versions of ourselves. Since losing your loved one, how have your views on grief changed?

Our responses to losing a loved one reveal hidden aspects of ourselves. We uncover strengths, more deeply understand our vulnerabilities, and lay bare our emotional cores. With this new understanding, we have a deeper sense of who we are, what we need, and what we would like to change. What has your grief taught you about yourself?

Unprepared for grief, we may wish others had told us what to expect, but at the same time we recognize that each person's experience is individual. Loss always comes with the unexpected. Writing out what we wish we had known about living with loss crystalizes our hard-earned knowledge. What would have helped you feel more prepared for grief?

WORK THROUGH THE UNEXPECTED

Grief is destabilizing. Unexpected situations, emotions, or revelations further upset stability. Identifying what has not changed, as well as reminding yourself that you can choose how to handle changes, helps return balance. Identify one or two unexpected aspects of grief that have been particularly difficult for you. What hasn't changed? What choices do you have? How do you want to handle it?

UNEXPECTED SITUATION/EMOTION

Partner's family doesn't talk to me

WAYS I CAN RESPOND

Get angry; ask why; ignore them; put energy into friends

WHY IS THIS DIFFICULT?

Felt abandoned by partner already; abandonment in childhood

WHAT HASN'T CHANGED

Strong friendships; partner's daughter still in my life

WEEK 39

The Many Meanings of Afterlife

MY LOVED ONE HAS AN AFTERLIFE IN MY MEMORIES AND IN THE STORIES I SHARE WITH OTHERS.

Our love doesn't stop with our loved one's death. One way of thinking about an afterlife is to consider how our dead live on, both in our memories and in the love we continue to feel for them. In what ways do you keep your loved one's memory alive?

Some will say our loved one is "in a better place." If we believe in an afterlife, this may be a comfort, though we still may prefer our loved ones to be here with us. If we believe nothing survives death, this reassurance can be offensive. How do you feel about a "better place"?

We are living a kind of afterlife, the life after the death of our loved ones. Though it can feel like no life at all or one that's been broken to bits, it is ours to live. This can be overwhelming. It feels impossible. Still, we persist. What is keeping you going this week?

Many of us were brought up with religious or cultural beliefs about life after death. Sometimes we carry these views throughout our lives. Other times we discard these beliefs or choose different ones. What did you learn about an afterlife growing up? What do you believe now?

VISUALIZE YOUR LOVED ONE

Even if you believe that life stops completely at death, it can be healing to envision your loved one free of the emotional pain or physical maladies they carried in life or experienced in their death. Take a few slow, deep breaths. Close your eyes if you wish and stop at any time if you become overwhelmed. Picture your loved one before you, liberated from all suffering. Their expression is vibrant, and they glow with health. Sit for a moment with your loved one, making eye contact with them. What do you notice? Do they speak to you or communicate in other ways? What would you like them to know? When you are ready, open your eyes.

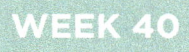

Love Survives Loss

I DRAW STRENGTH FROM MY LOVE FOR THE PERSON I GRIEVE. THIS LOVE IS ETERNAL AND CANNOT BE DESTROYED BY DEATH.

Love keeps us connected to our dead. It can make our grief more tolerable. Sometimes the love between us and those we've lost is complicated, particularly if our relationships were strained. Noting and acknowledging love's complications is another way to honor it. Is the love between you and the person you grieve complicated? If so, how?

When broken by grief and unable to go on, we can draw upon the love we received from those we've lost and hold ourselves in its warmth. Describe the love you and the person you lost shared. What was it like to be loved by them?

We cannot see love, but we can feel it, this invisible thread that links us to people we care about. It announces itself in our bodies, in rushes of warmth, in a pleasant ache in the chest. What do you feel in your body when you think about the love you shared with the person you lost?

It is possible to maintain a healthy love for and connection with the people we have lost. Sharing our memories about them is one way to do this. Living our lives fully post-loss in their honor is another. How do or will you maintain a connection to your loved one?

CREATE A SYMBOL OF YOUR LOVE

There are many symbols for love. Identify or create a symbol of love that is personal to you and your loved one. Think of something that represents the bond you share with the person you lost. This can come from a memory or significant object or can be more symbolic. For example, if you and your loved one liked to walk together, your love symbol might be something significant from your walks or a pair of hands intertwined. If you wish, include the difficulties attached to your love.

WEEK 41

Cultivating Gratitude

I AM GRATEFUL FOR THE TIME I SPENT WITH MY LOVED ONE AND FOR THE LOVE WE SHARED.

It can seem like a cruel joke to cultivate gratitude when our lives have been turned upside down. We don't want to be thankful. We just want our loved ones back. Still, gratitude affects the brain in positive ways and is beneficial for mental health. It could be worth a try. How do you feel about incorporating gratitude into your grief?

We honor our loved ones through our gratitude. Even when we struggle with feeling grateful in the wake of their deaths, we can recognize the positive ways they influenced us and the things about them we still carry. In what ways are you grateful for your loved one?

We've been through a lot, including death and its aftermath (and sometimes its precursors), the seemingly interminable grief, and the slow process of rebuilding our lives. Something within us persists and holds hope we will feel better. What are you grateful for in yourself?

Cultivating Gratitude

Recognizing those who have been there for us is another way to develop and nurture gratitude. Think of folks you are thankful for, looking to both your current life and the past. How have they been there for you? What would you like them to know?

ALLOW GRIEF AND GRATITUDE TO COEXIST

Gratitude is a necessary part of healing, but it doesn't alleviate the pain of grief. It makes it more bearable. Fill in the blanks to illustrate how your grief and gratitude coexist, using the example as a guide.

  I'm grateful for _____ but not for _____. I am thankful for _____ and feel _____. Although I feel gratitude for _____, I wish _____.

> **For example, I am grateful for** *my grandmother's presence in my childhood* **but not for** *how I saw her die in front of me.* **I am thankful for** *her love, which I have internalized* **and feel** *angry I was left without a protector.* **Although I feel gratitude for** *my happy memories of her,* **I wish** *she had lived until I was an adult.*

WEEK 42

Opening Up About Grief

**I HAVE THE RIGHT TO FEEL AND EXPRESS MY GRIEF.
BEING OPEN ABOUT MY FEELINGS NORMALIZES
GRIEF AND MAKES SPACE FOR HEALING.**

We may hide our sadness and suffering in the wake of loss, not wanting to feel judged or make others uncomfortable. Opening up about grief means allowing ourselves to be vulnerable. What would it look like if you were completely open about your feelings around your loss?

Some aspects of grief are hard to explain, so we keep them hidden. For example, we may grieve our sense of self or the future we thought we would have, in addition to missing our loved ones. Often there is no space to express these parts of our grief. Are there parts of your grief you keep hidden? Why?

Our comfort with sharing emotions depends on personality and privacy preferences. Although worries about being judged may be a factor in the decision to keep grief hidden, we may also feel more comfortable sharing our feelings with a trusted few or no one at all. How do your personality and sense of privacy affect how open you are about your grief?

Talking freely about grief helps us deal with it directly. When grief goes unspoken, it can appear as unhealthy habits, depression, and continued isolation. If there is no one we feel comfortable sharing with, joining a grief group or talking with a psychotherapist provides a safe space to express our feelings. Whom do you lean on for support around grief?

CHOOSE YOUR MOURNING SYMBOL

Mourning bands, usually black in color and worn around the upper arm, are public symbols of grief. You can create and wear your own symbol of grief, making it as public or private as you want. A loved one's ring, a meaningful piece of fabric, a token you keep in a pocket, and a tattoo can all be ways to mark your grief and remind you of your love. You can wear this symbol for a few months, a year, or forever. What would you choose as your symbol of mourning? Why?

WEEK 43

The Importance of Showing Up

I CHOOSE TO SHOW UP IN THE WORLD AUTHENTICALLY AND HONESTLY. WHEN I NEED A BREAK, I WILL TAKE IT.

After a loss, socializing can become overwhelming. We may disengage from social contact because it takes too much energy. Eventually, however, we need to rejoin the world or risk being stuck in our grief. What comes up for you when you think about reengaging in life?

Grief undermines our belief in ourselves and our interest in life. With our loved ones gone, existence feels gray and dull. Showing up can feel unimportant and irrelevant. It takes extra effort to spark our motivation. What motivates you to show up? What gets in the way?

_____

_____

_____

_____

_____

_____

We may be keeping up socially but also keeping grief hidden. Continuing to conceal our pain contributes to loneliness and isolation, even when we show up in other ways. Sharing our grief with others helps us show up authentically and feel less alone. Are you hiding your grief? What would it be like to be more open about your feelings?

_____

_____

_____

_____

_____

_____

For the first year after my father's death, my stepmother made a point to say "yes" to all invitations. Travel groups, visits with friends, and excursions to the city led to new friendships and experiences. When could you say "yes," even when it is difficult to show up?

GROUND YOURSELF

The mountain pose is a simple yoga position. It can help you feel grounded, providing a foundation for showing up in the world. Stand with your bare feet together or hip-width apart, whichever is most comfortable for you, with your weight evenly distributed. Keep your knees soft. Lengthen your spine and neck, tucking your chin slightly. Leave your arms by your sides with your hands relaxed or fingers spread out, or bring your hands together at the center of your chest. Feel your connection to the earth, your feet like the mountain foothills, your head the mountain's peak. Breathe deeply, your chest expanding as you feel steady and rooted. Use this pose to ground you before going to social events or other activities that feel daunting.

WEEK 44

Finding Strength in Yourself and Others

I DRAW UPON MY INNER STRENGTH, FRIENDS AND FAMILY, AND COMMUNITY TO SUPPORT ME AFTER LOSS.

When our internal resources are stretched to the limit, having other sources of strength to call upon helps us through. These can be friends, healing spaces, or rituals and practices that keep us going when it seems we can't go on. What other resources can you call upon when your strength is flagging?

Self-care after loss includes identifying online or print resources for support. Searching a therapist directory, signing up for an online grief support group, and checking out the self-help section at the bookstore are all ways we can take care of ourselves. How have you used these resources to support you in grief?

I've gotten through many difficult periods, including times of grief, using humor to cope. Humor helps distract us from our pain. When we can use that pain as a source for humor, we create something joyful out of suffering. How do you use humor to help you with loss?

Sometimes we need to create something or move our bodies to cultivate joy and rejuvenate ourselves. Dancing or singing may be ways to nurture the spark within. Creating a delicious meal and writing a poem are other approaches. How can you cultivate joy and rejuvenate yourself when your internal resources are spent?

IDENTIFY YOUR STRENGTHS

Identifying and writing down your strengths will help you recognize and draw upon them during grief's tough times. Write two to three positive things about yourself in each category. For example, you may have met the challenge of speaking up in a difficult work environment, developed the skill of deep listening, valued kindness, and learned how to take feedback. Perhaps you had to make a tough decision to leave a relationship and others see you as honest. Return to this list when you need to remind yourself of the power you hold within.

CHALLENGES I'VE MET

_____

_____

_____

MY TALENTS AND SKILLS

_____

_____

_____

MY VALUES

_____

_____

_____

LESSONS I'VE LEARNED

_____

_____

_____

TOUGH DECISIONS I'VE MADE

_____

_____

_____

WHAT OTHERS SEE IN ME

_____

_____

_____

WEEK 45

Handling the Permanence of Loss

WHEN IT FEELS IMPOSSIBLE TO ENDURE MY LOVED ONE'S ABSENCE, I REMIND MYSELF THAT I CARRY THEM WITH ME.

Grief gives us an unendurable task that we have no choice but to endure—to live without our loved ones until we ourselves are gone. The permanence of their absence gets heavier with the passage of time. How do you endure this fact of loss?

Some of us like to imagine our loved ones here with us always. Others are more comfortable separating from their memories, keeping their relationships in the past, making them things of occasional reverie. Are you drawn to holding your loved one close or letting them go? Why?

Knowing we carry aspects of our loved ones with us in memory, stories, and love isn't the same as having them here in flesh and blood. It's all we've got, but it doesn't always feel like enough. How do you get through the days when you miss your loved one so much it hurts?

Sometimes I imagine myself surrounded by the pets and people I've lost. We're a congenial, rumpled bunch, a chaotic group catching up at a homey house party. This fantasy lets me bring my dead back to life. What fantasies do you have about spending time with your loved one?

_____
_____
_____
_____
_____
_____
_____

CALM YOURSELF WITH BUTTERFLY TAPPING

Sometimes called a butterfly hug, butterfly tapping is a therapy technique that can help you feel grounded during those times when you miss your loved one with a painful intensity. Alternating taps between each side of the body, also known as bilateral stimulation, helps calm anxiety, and butterfly tapping is an easy way to do this. Start by crossing your hands palms down on your chest, interlocking your thumbs and fanning out your fingers. Your fingers should be pointed toward your neck, with the tip of the middle finger just below the collarbone. Tap one hand and then the other, slowly trading taps back and forth, as though your hands were the slowly beating wings of a butterfly. Continue tapping for at least thirty seconds. If butterfly tapping is difficult, other forms of bilateral stimulation, such as moving your eyes back and forth, alternating taps on your thighs, or shifting weight from one foot to the other can also work.

WEEK 46

Creating Meaning and Finding Purpose

I WILL CREATE A MEANINGFUL, PURPOSEFUL LIFE TO HONOR BOTH MYSELF AND MY LOVED ONE.

Making meaning and finding purpose are lifelong endeavors that require flexibility and self-compassion. When death has pushed us off course and mangled any sense of meaning, it can be helpful to remember other times when we've had to create a meaningful life after a change. Write about a previous time you had to create meaning out of difficult circumstances.

Death removes our sense of purpose, robbing our lives of meaning and limiting our capacities to create it. Sadness, fear, and numbness can keep us frozen in place. We may want to create meaning but feel unsure of how or whether that is possible. What might get in the way of creating meaning after your loss?

Grief expert David Kessler called making meaning the sixth stage of grief, an essential part of integrating the deaths of our loved ones into our lives. Navigating this sixth stage involves letting our love for those we've lost outweigh the pain of their absences. It also means using our lives to honor our loved ones. How will you approach the sixth stage of grief?

Creating Meaning and Finding Purpose

Taking on someone's positive qualities, organizing for a cause in their name, and using their love as a foundation for a meaningful life are all ways to create meaning and purpose out of loss. How can you use your loved one's life or death to help you create meaning and purpose for yourself?

PLAN A MEANINGFUL FUTURE

Like an earthquake, your loved one's death shifted the ground underneath you, upending your purpose. As you start to rebuild, you can use what you valued about your life with your loved one to create a purposeful plan for a meaningful future. Use the following categories to create a structure. For example, I had someone who really listened to me. I value the art of deep listening, and I plan to become a better listener.

WHAT I HAD WITH MY LOVED ONE

PLAN FOR THE FUTURE

WHAT I VALUE

WEEK 47

Giving Back

I SHARE MY LIGHT, NURTURE MY HEART, AND HONOR MY LOVED ONE BY HELPING OTHERS.

Helping others helps us transcend our grief and create something positive out of loss. This help can take many forms, from supporting fellow grievers to volunteering at an organization our loved one supported or contributing time to an important cause. Altruism and volunteer work do not come naturally to everyone. What are your thoughts and feelings about devoting time or resources to helping others?

We can show up for others in small ways, such as bringing food to an ill friend or listening deeply to another grieving person. These small acts of presence are good for other people as well as for us. In what small ways do you help others? How do these actions make you feel?

Sharing our wounded places is a daunting exercise in vulnerability. Exposing our emotional scars and tender spots to people who have been through similar experiences helps us feel less alone. The shared experience of vulnerability connects us. What comes up for you when you imagine being vulnerable around your experiences with loss?

Joining a group for grievers allows us to support others and also be supported by them. We take comfort in acceptance and shared experience. Even though each person's grief is personal to them, we recognize places of overlap. What do you think about grief groups? If you have participated in a group, what was the experience like?

_____
_____
_____
_____
_____
_____
_____
_____
_____

FIND VOLUNTEER OPPORTUNITIES

Even if you are not yet ready to or are not interested in volunteering, it can be inspiring to see the opportunities available. This exercise opens a space to learn more about available volunteer and other support positions. VolunteerMatch.org is a good resource for finding virtual and in-person general volunteer work near you. If you want to get involved in grief-related volunteering, search your local area for hospices and organizations that assist the bereaved. Think about what interests you and on a separate piece of paper list potential ways you could help others. Include specific opportunities you have identified through VolunteerMatch.org or other resources.

WEEK 48

Checking in with Where You Are Now

AS I PROCESS MY GRIEF, MY FEELINGS SHIFT AND CHANGE. I RECOGNIZE MY CAPACITY TO GROW AND ADAPT.

Over time, our relationship with grief changes. Things that felt impossible to overcome are no longer difficult. Situations that seemed less fraught in the early days have become harder to navigate. Consider how your grief has shifted in the past six months. What has become harder? What is easier?

Although it can be tricky to have specific expectations of our grieving process, letting go of all expectations is frustrating and unhelpful. At the same time, we quickly become discouraged when it seems like we are stuck in grief. How do you balance a desire for progress with the unpredictable nature of loss?

Some aspects of grief may remain stable as time passes. This happens for a variety of reasons. We may, for example, not want things to change. We also could feel stuck or struggle with moving forward, perhaps out of guilt or difficulty relinquishing our loved one. In what ways has your grief remained the same? Why?

We recognize and meet loss's challenges and see its unpredictable nature at work in our lives. These experiences help us anticipate how we will weather our grief over time. Consider what you know about living with loss. What words of encouragement do you have for yourself as you continue to live with grief?

REWORK PROMPTS TO MARK CHANGE

Each response to a prompt is a snapshot of your grieving process over time. Looking back through old prompts and writing new responses from your current viewpoint helps you recognize how you and your grief have changed over time. Look back through previous weeks to identify prompts that were particularly meaningful or difficult. You could also choose prompts that resonate with you now.

Checking in with Where You Are Now

WEEK 49

Finding Comfort in Beauty

I NOTICE BEAUTY ALL AROUND, IN THE UNFURLING SPRING LEAVES, IN THE KINDNESS OF FRIENDS, IN THE SUNLIGHT THROUGH MY WINDOW.

In the black and gray world curated by grief, beauty is elusive. Often, we are not yet ready to notice beauty or are so dulled by grief that we don't see it in front of us. Will we ever see beauty again? What are your feelings, fears, and hopes about finding beauty after loss?

Because our loved ones can no longer take pleasure in lovely things, our own enjoyment can seem wrong. We feel guilty for our aliveness and cut ourselves off from the world's beauty. But it is possible that our appreciation of beauty honors those we have lost. Do you agree? Disagree? Why?

"Beauty," Shakespeare wrote, "is bought by judgment of the eye." What we find beautiful is subjective and not limited to the things we can see or visualize. We can experience beauty in a song, a touch, a delicious meal, or community with others. Where do you find beauty?

Grief gives us no choice but to feel it or feel numb. We can't sprint through its sludge of sadness, loneliness, and regret. Grieving takes time because it comes from a deep, wounded, and yet connected place. The ache is a profound, and perhaps beautiful, sign of our capacity to love. Do you see beauty in your grief? How?

CONNECT WITH BEAUTY

Visit a place you find beautiful. It can be a mountain trail, a museum, or your backyard, anywhere beautiful to you. If you cannot visit in person, use a picture or video for inspiration. Go to this place and let your senses take it in, then write down your impressions when you are done. Notice the sounds around you and the fragrances carried in the air. What colors do you see? Is the air dry or saturated? What textures can you feel? Are plants and animals in this place? People? What do they look like? How does it feel to be in this place?

WEEK 50

Recognizing Your Inner Strength

I AM STRONG AND POWERFUL. I WEATHER MY GRIEF, MOVE FORWARD WHEN I FEEL STUCK, AND HOLD HOPE FOR MY FUTURE.

Much like we can appreciate our loved ones for who they were, imperfections and all, we can appreciate ourselves as we are, human and fallible. This can be difficult if we are perfectionists. Are there ways that you expect perfection from yourself as a griever? Where could you use a little self-compassion?

Change comes in small steps. It can show up in how we approach and experience the stuck times and temporary setbacks of grief. Learning how to weather the ups and downs of our grieving processes is an important part of integrating our losses into our lives. How has your capacity to handle grief's pitfalls changed over time?

_____

_____

_____

_____

_____

_____

Applauding others may come naturally to us, but identifying our own progress can be difficult, which makes seeing how far we've come challenging. Imagine you could see yourself from the viewpoint of a close friend or your loved one. What would they say about how far you've come since your loss?

_____

_____

_____

_____

_____

_____

Sometimes we can use what we consider our flaws to our advantage. Stubbornness can be helpful in situations where we need to press on. A skeptical nature sometimes keeps us from being taken advantage of. Being obsessive about details is essential when details are vital. How have your flaws been advantageous as you navigate grief and your post-loss life?

_____

_____

_____

_____

_____

_____

_____

_____

HONOR YOUR CAPACITY TO SURVIVE

Something within you keeps you going after loss. Spend a moment to picture this strong, survival-oriented part of you. Is it hard and multifaceted, like a diamond? Is it a creature that is both soft and sharp, like a cat with claws bared? Or perhaps this part is human in nature, strong, silent, and aware, walking softly but carrying a big stick. Where do you hold this part of you in your body? Is it heart, head, or gut focused? Would you describe it as more a thinking and perceiving part, a sort of watchfulness, or more a feeling, intuitive part acting on instinct? Give this part a name.

WEEK 51

What Does It Mean to Heal?

MY HEALING IS A PROCESS. AS I HEAL AND GROW, I AM GRATEFUL FOR MY TIME WITH MY LOVED ONE.

We may feel that healing completely after loss is impossible. Or perhaps we hope for healing but are not sure what it looks like. What does healing after your loss mean to you?

When we get caught up in our loved ones' deaths, we often ignore their lives. Sad endings overshadow happy memories. Healing may include allowing our loved ones' lives to matter more than their deaths. This can take time. Where are you in this part of your healing?

_____
_____
_____
_____
_____
_____

We may sometimes wish we had never met our loved ones. All this pain and endless processing wouldn't have been necessary if we'd never crossed paths. But that would have meant missing out on knowing and being known by them. Holding pain and love simultaneously is part of healing. Describe how you hold the pain of loss alongside love.

_____
_____
_____
_____
_____
_____

Healing requires self-care and self-compassion. Taking care of the basics, such as getting enough food and rest, is important. But there are other activities that are also vital. For example, reading fiction keeps me on an even keel and supports my healing. What supports your healing?

REPRESENT YOUR HEALING IN COLORS

Recognizing that our feelings after loss vary and change is part of living with grief. This exercise provides a visual representation of the healing process.

Using the following list, choose a different color for each emotion you've experienced, crossing out emotions that don't fit and adding ones that do. On a separate sheet of paper, draw a circle and divide it into multiple sections, each corresponding to a time range. For example, to represent a year of grief, you could divide the circle into four sections, each corresponding to three months. Label the sections and color in each period with the emotions you experienced in proportion to their intensity. For example, if you were particularly shocked, anxious, and angry in one period, use more of those colors to fill in that section. Compare the sections to see how your grief has shifted over time. Redo this exercise periodically to see what has changed.

Shock	**Loneliness**
Anger	**Fear**
Sadness	**Hope**
Love	**Relief**
Guilt	**Anxiety**

WEEK 52

Visualizing the Future

**I LOOK FORWARD TO THE FUTURE AND TO CREATING
A LIFE FULL OF CONNECTION AND MEANING.**

In the immediate aftermath of death and loss, the future can look unclear or feel nonexistent. Investing in a future post-loss may mean letting go of the life we wish we had, but it is a necessary part of healing. What does it mean for you to anticipate and plan for a future?

Not everything changes after a loss. The core of who we are, the people we are close to, or our communities may remain stable. Noting what has and will stay the same helps us feel grounded as we consider the future. What will remain stable for you going forward?

As time goes on, we will continue to hold space for those we've lost, integrating their memories into our lives. Each of us will approach this in different ways, from regular cemetery visits to having daily conversations with our loved ones. How will you make a place for your grief in the future?

Envisioning a future means integrating the past. Imagine your life as a series of books. One volume is devoted to the time before your loss. Another encompasses your grief up to the present. The third book represents your future. What would you title these three volumes?

CREATE INTENTIONS FOR THE FUTURE

Creating intentions mindfully can help you see them to fruition. Begin by focusing on what you'd like to do and why. From there, create specific steps to follow through with. As you continue to heal and process your grief, what would you like more of in your life? What aligns with your values? What will help you make your intentions reality? Write two intentions for the future, using the example as a guide.

WHAT I WANT MORE OF IN MY LIFE

I want to connect more with friends.

WHY?

I value friendship. When I feel connected, I am also happier and less lonely.

STEPS I WILL TAKE

I will seek out groups focused on [activity] by [date]. I will also reach out to [friend] by phone, text, or email by [date].

RESOURCES

Books

Cacciatore, Joanne, PhD. *Bearing the Unbearable: Love, Loss, and the Heartbreaking Path of Grief*.
Guidance on living with traumatic loss

Devine, Megan. *It's OK That You're Not OK: Meeting Grief and Loss in a Culture That Doesn't Understand*.
Personal experience with traumatic loss and support for others going through it

Didion, Joan. *The Year of Magical Thinking*.
Nonfiction chronicle of the first year after a husband's sudden death

Helbert, Karla. *Yoga for Grief and Loss*.
How to use yoga and associated practices to process grief

Rando, Therese A., PhD. *How to Go on Living When Someone You Love Dies*.
Comprehensive, practical guide about what to do after loss

Websites

Dougy Center
Dougy.org
Grief support for children, teens, young adults, and their families

Modern Loss
ModernLoss.com
Grief-related personal essays, resources, and articles

National Suicide Prevention Lifeline
1-800-273-8255
SuicidePreventionLifeline.org
Free, confidential emotional support for people in suicidal or emotional crisis

Online support groups and live chat for grievers
Grieving.com
Variety of support groups run by peers

Open Path Psychotherapy Collective
OpenPathCollective.org
Nonprofit, nationwide network of mental health professionals who offer affordable psychotherapy

Professional Support, Online Groups, and Hotlines

Grief in Common
GriefinCommon.com

SAMHSA Behavioral Health Services Locator
1-800-662-HELP (4357)
FindTreatment.samhsa.gov
Free, confidential service provided by the federal Substance Abuse and Mental Health Services Administration

Survivors of Violent Loss Network
SVLP.org
Support and information for those who have lost someone to violence

The Compassionate Friends
CompassionateFriends.org
Resources and support after the loss of a child

The Dinner Party
TheDinnerParty.org
Community for grieving 20- and 30-somethings

Therapy Den
TherapyDen.com
Nationwide, inclusive directory of psychotherapists

Acknowledgments

Writing this book coincided with a serious health issue in my family as well as with the death of a beloved pet. I am grateful to my husband and son for providing me the space to write and continue my work during a destabilizing time. Navigating a new health landscape, and at the same time working, going to school, taking care of our home and our remaining pets, and reading my drafts is no small feat. I also am grateful to my mother for instilling in me a love of language and precision with words and to my stepmother for providing an authentic, loving example of how to grieve. I couldn't have written a thing without any of you. Thank you.

About the Author

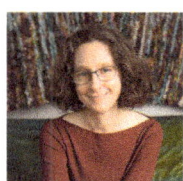

JENNIFER TRINKLE, LMFT, is a licensed psychotherapist and former librarian. She lives in the San Francisco Bay Area with her family, cats, greyhound, and galgo. This is her first book.

Printed in the USA
CPSIA information can be obtained
at www.ICGtesting.com
JSHW070829080224
56755JS00009B/97